TRIBE OF MEN

TRIBE OF MEN

MICHAEL KING

NEW DEGREE PRESS

COPYRIGHT © 2021 MICHAEL KING

All rights reserved.

TRIBE OF MEN

ISBN   978-1-63730-808-0 *Paperback*
             978-1-63730-867-7 *Kindle Ebook*
             978-1-63730-980-3 *Ebook*

CONTENTS

———

INTRODUCTION

In the world we live in today, there exists a gender of the human race which is largely misunderstood, misinterpreted, and judged. Men have, for centuries, been tossed here and there between definitions and varying expectations, and for the most part of it, the definition of who a good man is varies all the time. A lot of men suffer from depression, anxiety disorders—the list goes on. It's a sad fact we've had to hide our issues in a bid to preserve a false picture of masculinity. Being a man or trying to live up to the proverbial tough stereotype doesn't always solve the problem. The issues we face as men are real and tangible. Real issues need real solutions—not philosophical or psuedo-inspirational suggestions but a clear manual that will aid our journey through the struggles we face daily and the societal pressures that constantly surround us.

It's a constant battle, and many things try to drive you crazy at the same time. There is an enemy we see in the form of opposition from people to circumstances and situations we find ourselves in. The most critical battle arena is not when we encounter these persons and situations but in the battlefield of the mind. Once a man loses his mental battle, he'll surely lose the physical ones. This is simply because whatever happens upstairs determines the course of your life. Securing your mental health is no joke. It doesn't make you a sissy; rather, it makes you smart. If the mind is such an important influence on your chance for success, why should you play with it?

There's a movement of men changing the emotionless man script, and stats suggest now is the time for men to find healthy outlets for their stress. Did you know?

- Current stats suggest one out of three men regularly feel lonely.
- About 30.6 percent of men have suffered from a period of depression in their lifetime according to a 2013 study from the Journal of American Medical Association. The number of males affected by depression per year is six million, according to Mental Health America.
- Low levels of testosterone are correlated with depression, stress, and mood swings, especially among older men.
- One in five adults experience mental health problems each year with serious mental illness costing Americans $193.2 billion in lost earnings per year.

Despite these shocking numbers, it is still taboo for men to speak openly about their mental health. Anger, anxiety, lack of hope, lack of purpose, and no plan for growth and development can be a breeding ground for depression for some men. However, topics like loneliness, worrying, sadness, moody behavior, relationship challenges, abuse, and trauma are real-life issues a lot of men hide because they don't want to appear weak.

The old saying goes, "You can't teach an old dog new tricks," but this isn't true for dogs or humans. We are products of our environment, so exposure to new environments and ways of thinking may be the key to unlearning the toxic, ineffective thoughts and behaviors that are unproductive. Toxic men sparked the #MeToo movement, empowering women to speak up against the abuse experienced as a result of dark side of masculinity. The male code causes some men to never feel like they fit in, and they are seeking a way to be their authentic selves. Some men live a life feeling empty without finding their purpose.

This book is not about broken hearts or lost dreams. It's about rebounding from adversity, breaking out of the man box, normalizing therapy for men, and the movement to evolve masculinity for the good of all. Guys, if unmet expectations have you feeling discouraged and having a sour outlook on life, if you're tired of struggling to find your purpose in life, bogged down by feelings of insignificance. Then this book is for you. Men who feel like they're stuck in the rat race of life, who feel like they repeat patterns from failed relationships, who fall into the traps of addiction, anxiety, isolation, depression, and patterns of poverty mind-set. At times, do you feel like your career and personal development is fizzling under the pressures of being an adult? This book is your guide to value your mental health and wellness to become emotionally intelligent, secure, and relationship ready.

Great men are not born, they are forged in the furnace of adversity. When life turns on the heat, we must respond and not overreact. I remember a saying I once heard that a carpenter often thinks he can solve all his problems with a hammer. But some problems can't be solved by the regular means we are used to. Having the right knowledge provides you with the tools that will help you respond properly in any situation. This book is focused on healing, care, and faith. It is garnished with the ingredients of greatness. It doesn't matter where this book finds you or where you found this book, all that matters is you and the great potentials that are embedded deep within. With this book in your hand, you'll never need to walk alone.

Let's go!

CHAPTER 1

MEN NEED
SELF-CARE TOO!

WHAT EXACTLY DOES SELF-CARE MEAN TO YOU?
Close your eyes and think about that question for a few minutes. Does a picture come to mind? Surely you can come up with a few scenarios and examples that would describe what self-care means to you. Is it a profound nap? A warm bath after a hard day's work? Getting your hair done? Seeing a movie? A vacation?

Whatever it is you picture to be an ideal self-care activity, it is very probable to assume you also imagined a woman engaging in said activity. Does that mean men do not need self-care too? Before we examine that question, let's take a look at what self-care means.

Essentially, self-care is just a blanket term that encapsulates a set of activities, rituals, and other practices (however simple or complex you want yours to be) people engage in to help recharge, refresh, and re-center themselves again.

These activities enhance a person's happiness and general well-being.

One thing most people don't take into consideration about self-care is the fact it goes beyond just resting and pampering yourself. Self-care takes a lot of work and time and as such, requires a certain level of dedication. This would make certain the purpose of engaging in said activity is not defeated.

WHAT'S IN IT FOR MEN?

Self-care is just as important to the well-being of all people. Most men are not open to the idea of taking time for themselves. The reason for this is how society has made it look like men do not need to take breaks and it is effeminate for men to open up to other people about their personal struggles, as they should face their problems "like a man." The general idea of a man is one who works day in and day out and does not need to take breaks. However, this state of mind is inconsistent with reality.

Men experience burnouts too. Strokes and other blood pressure issues, which are prevalent among men, can be attributed to a lack of self-care. Most men, being too busy with work and raising and taking care of a family (that most times may include members of their extended families too), do not think they need to make time to take care of themselves. The result of this is men are beginning to burn out faster. High blood pressure and other illnesses that used to be considered "old people illnesses" have begun to affect young and middle-aged men too. The pressure society continues to pile upon men to live up to a certain standard of "manliness" is about to plunge the male population into one health issue or another and has already begun to decrease the life expectancy of men in most countries.

Men need to understand self-care is just as important to them as they perceive it to be in the case of women. Every man, no matter how busy they think themselves to be, should endeavor to take some time and engage in activities that would help them unwind and keep them refreshed and rejuvenated. Here are a few examples of activities \ every man should take time to periodically engage in:

HIT THE GYM

Exercising is one of the best self-care practices a man should be actively engaged in. Exercising every day, or at least once every other day, should be a constant feature in every man's life, no matter how busy they think they are. If the nature of your job demands you cannot go to the gym every day, you can wake up early and jog a certain distance around your area of residence. If that is not a safe practice, due to the security level in your neighborhood, you can still do a couple push-ups before heading out for work. Then you can go to the gym during the weekend, if you can afford a gym subscription. If not, you should at least jog in the evenings or take strolls.

The advantages of engaging in physical exercise include higher self-esteem, better sleep, as well as less feelings of depression and anxiety. Any time you engage in physical exercises, your body releases endorphins that trigger a feel-good sensation just like morphine. This motivates the body to keep going on its path to peak physical health and shape (Bruce 2020).

EAT HEALTHY

Most men do not give much thought to their nutrition. Unhealthy eating practices such as drinking carbonated drinks, not eating enough fruits and vegetables, et cetera are common among men. As a man, you should understand your body is only as strong and healthy as what you feed it. You must therefore make sure to eat food that is rich in nutrients. Eggs, fruits, and vegetables, et cetera are necessary for the sufficient supply of proteins and vitamins, which are required to keep your body from unnecessary breakdown due to stress. Foods rich in calories are also needed to supply the much-needed energy that goes into all of that hard work you do.

START JOURNALING

Journaling means writing down or documenting events and happenings (positive, in this case). No matter what hobbies you decide to take on as a part of your self-care regimen, every man should make journaling a habit. The form you choose to make your journal in does not matter.

The idea is to consciously search for and seek out positive things (met goals and achievements, as well as other things to be grateful for). Over time, this habit makes you perceive your life differently and gives you an outlook of life that is mostly positive. Journaling not only makes you a more intro-spective man but also makes you accountable to yourself by giving you the space to write down your goals and keep track of your progress in the course of achieving these goals.

RECITE AFFIRMATIONS

A lot of people think affirmations are a tired joke at best. They do not understand how saying a couple words could impact your life in any way. You must not become one of these people. Affirmations are positive statements that help you rewire your mind and overcome self-sabotaging, negative thoughts. These positive statements permeate our conscious and subconscious minds to reprogram our thought patterns.

A great feature of affirmations is the fact they can be tailored to fit our various personal preferences. Some people prefer to create their own affirmations, which is what I would recommend, as they would be better phrased to suit the particular purpose for which you made your affirmation in the first place. Others prefer guided affirmations which can be found on YouTube. Whatever approach works best for you, affirmations are an ideal addition to your self-care routine and should be followed through consecutively for thirty days at least to experience a change in your mind-set.

ENHANCE YOUR SPIRITUALITY

Take some time to meditate every day. Find a quiet spot in your house and spend a few hours every day speaking to God and speaking kindly to your own subconscious self. Speak to God as you would speak to someone you trust. Confide in him and allow him to take away all of the emotional burden you had been bearing and trust he has your best intentions on his mind. Attend church service. Give to the needy and to charitable causes. All of these activities will begin to foster a feeling of oneness with the universe. You will also begin to feel at peace with the world you live in, which in turn enhances your sense of self as well as your general well-being as a man.

Besides the points we have already examined, there are countless other numerous self-care activities every man should indulge in. Here are a few examples of some smaller ideas I have found helpful in my own journey:

Get off your screen! Read a book: Every day. Besides broadening your scope of thought and shaping your world view as a man, reading can also be calming. You can pick an hour each day and read a book. Better still, make it a part of your night routine. Just before you sleep, you can read a book for fifteen to thirty minutes to calm your system and bring yourself to sleep.

Take Walks: This is another massively underrated self-care activity. Walks bring you into contact with nature as well as allowing you to be by yourself enough to unclutter your mind and develop new perspectives about things. Your walks should be just long enough to let you connect with nature and take in its essence. You should also be able to think things through with the enhanced mental clarity the walk would provide you with. This little bit of exercise in combination with clearing your head can offer a great deal of wellness.

Love yourself: Yes, I know. It doesn't exactly sound like "manly" advice. It isn't either. Self-love is a habit every human being, male or female, should endeavor to cultivate. Buy yourself clothing from time to time. Get a haircut. Get a manicure or pedicure (as frequently as you can afford to). Talk kindly to yourself. Listen to music that lifts your spirits. Make a conscious effort to be happy. All of these actions are guaranteed to enhance your general well-being as a man and draw people to you naturally.

Spend time with people that value you: Your energy and sense of self-worth are some of your greatest driving forces as a man. As such, you should be careful about the kind of people who you choose to spend time with. INTENTIONALITY is the watchword here. Everything about your interactions with other people must be intentional. Nothing about the kind and quality of friendships you keep as a man should be left to chance. This is because the quality of the company you keep can make or mar you.

Make sure to avoid spending time with people who make you feel less of a man than you ought to. People who feel the need to talk you down do not deserve a place in your life, as they will continually attempt to chip away at your self-confidence until you begin to lose faith in your ability to achieve your personal goals and objectives.

Stop hanging out with people who do not have any long-term goals for their lives. This is because their *lassiez-faire* attitude to things could influence you and ultimately deter you from chasing and achieving your own goals.

Spend time with people who value and respect you. People who support your ambition and are constantly rooting for you to succeed are the people who you should spend quality time with. That does not translate to always hanging out with "yes-men" and people who will always tell you what they think you want to hear; these people will only be in your life for the furtherance of their own personal gain. They will not hesitate to jump ship once things start to go south with you.

Spend time with people who are honest with you—people who will not shy away from calling you out whenever you make a misstep. These are the only kind of people who you should let into your life.

MAYBE GET INTO SKINCARE?

Most men assume skincare is just for women. This could not be any further from the truth. Start using essential oils on your skin. Pick a scent you agree with and enhance your presence anywhere you go to with a great cologne and clear skin.

The bottom line is this: Do away with the idea you do not need to make time for some self-care or rely on others to be responsible for you as a man. Men need self-care too. Starting today, please go out of your way to take care of yourself. Don't wait until you burn out or fall sick before going to have your health status checked. Don't wait until you're about to meet someone to smell nice. Practice personal hygiene for your own personal well-being and not to impress people. Prioritize taking care of yourself, and your health will thank you for it because men need self-care too.

CHAPTER 2

BUILDING SOLID RELATIONSHIPS

———

We all maintain more than a few relationships on different levels. You literally cannot coexist on this planet with other people and not relate with them, however distant and remote the nature of your contact with them is. From total strangers who you encounter every day in the course of your day-to-day activity to your immediate family, friends, spouses, et cetera. As a man, your level of commitment and duties to people differ according to the nature of relationship you maintain with them.

Your responsibilities to your parents are very much different from your spousal duties to your partner. Your relationship with your friends surely cannot be of the same nature as your relationship with your children. Making all of these relationships work would require a certain level of commitment from you, as the man, to be there for the people who you keep these relationships with. You must commit to becoming a better man for your family, your friends, et cetera. As utopian and out of reach as the idea sounds, being a better man is not as difficult or unrealistically demanding as one might think. It all boils down to refining your character, both as a partner and as an individual. Here are a few ways to be a truly better man, for those around you:

EXPRESS YOURSELF

You cannot afford to continue bottling up things that bother you in the name of "being a man." The days when men kept everything to themselves to the point they broke from the inside are long gone. The consequences of not finding a healthy outlet to express and talk about the way you feel, as a man, are a lot graver than any shame you might be feeling about speaking to someone about the way you feel. It is not even a manly trait to avoid confrontations whether they be with people or circumstances. The "be a man" saying should be understood to translate to confronting your problems head-on and working to fix them by any means practicable.

Your relationships will suffer greatly if you continue to try to bear down upon your worries and try to handle things by yourself. Your love life will suffer, as you will grow more and more emotionally unavailable to your partner. This could potentially strain your relationship with them. Your friendships could potentially get strained as well. Your friends would definitely notice a change in your behavior and mood. They would try to reach out, and if you kept shutting them out, they might decide to leave entirely. Your relationships with your colleagues at work could also potentially be affected as well. Bottling up emotions for long enough can affect workplace output as well as your conduct at work.

The truth is the more expressive a man is about his feelings, the more genuine he is as a partner. If you feel sad, cry it out! If you feel annoyed, say it! If you feel thrilled, show it! If you express yourself, your partner, friends, colleagues, and every other person who you have cause to come in contact with will not only appreciate your openness but will also be open to effectively help you deal with whatever it is you're going through. They get to know the real you as opposed to the facade you put up when you ignore and push your emotions to the side.

TAKE A PAUSE AND LISTEN

Listening goes beyond just hearing what the other person is saying. It is an entire art form you should endeavor to master. You need to have the ability to not only hear what others are saying but also to understand what they mean. You should be able to react to what they are saying without interjecting your own position unless invited to do so. Listening skills could definitely take a while to get a firm grip on. However, the enhancement in the quality of your relationships would be a worthwhile reward for the commitment you had to put into being a better listener. Listening greatly benefits both parties; your partner gets a confidant to whom they can openly express their thoughts, and you gain an awareness about what is going through your partner's mind allowing you to comfort them better. The same goes for your friends and your children too. They learn they can trust you and you value them enough to listen to their concerns and triumphs, as well as their fears. Therefore, endeavor to always listen.

BE SUPPORTIVE

Support goes a long way, especially in relationships. As a man, you should make an effort to be there for the people who matter to you whenever they face any setbacks. The same applies as well for every milestone they reach. Celebrate with them too. For every new dream they share with you, dream with them! Make constructive inputs wherever you can and always let them understand through your words as well as your actions you will continually be there for them. The more you show your support, the more your partner, friends, and family will look to you as the right person to fall and stand up with. Much like trust, the more you give, the more you receive.

ACCEPT AND RESPECT YOUR PARTNER'S PREFERENCES

This point relates to your relationship with your spouse. Just because you're their soul mate doesn't mean you have to share their opinions and ideas on everything. By any criteria, that is not a reasonable expectation. You and your partner will almost certainly disagree on something, whether it's politics, religion, music, smartphone brand, or fashion. Unless your partner's interests are blatantly damaging or dangerous, you must learn to tolerate and appreciate their variations in preferences.

SURPRISE TO ADD SPICE

Relationships grow routine, stale, and eventually die the moment we begin to relax and stop working on them. This is especially true for couples who have been together for an extended period of time. Surprise your sweetheart every now and then to keep the relationship fresh. Prepare a surprise supper for her when she returns home; tuck a love letter into her luggage before she leaves for work; or organize a surprise vacation for the two of you! You might go for a big surprise or a small one, but what counts is it renews your bond. Be sneaky and inventive!

GIVE AND MAKE TIME

Time is an immensely valuable asset of yours as a man; this is because it is a finite commodity that can only be spent once. Giving and creating time for your partner is a clear sign you truly care about them. A hectic schedule, on the other hand, can make this difficult, but when things get tough, you have to work even harder. It doesn't have to be long all of the time. A shared lunch or a phone call may suffice, or, in the worst-case scenario, a promise to be available on a specific date may be adequate. What is important is you devote some of your time to your partner on a regular basis.

Make them feel important to you. No matter how tight your schedule may be, you can always find a way to take out a few twenty-five to thirty minutes once a week at least to spend with your partner. When you do get to be with them, give them your full attention. Switch off your mobile phone or put it on silent mode so it does not distract you. Be interested in what is happening in their life. Basically, be present. Don't be the kind of man who checks his phone every other minute while he is supposed to be spending some quality time with his partner. It's not just rude and disrespectful, but also speaks to how much that moment (and by extension, the relationship with your partner) matters to you.

TRUST AND BE TRUSTWORTHY

Without a shadow of doubt, one of the most vital components of a long-lasting relationship is trust. As a result, it's only natural for a man in any relationship to learn not only to trust his girlfriend but also to be someone worth trusting. If your partner goes to a party with her pals, don't be the guy who immediately suspects she'll be up to anything bad. You should trust her and her love for you if you know her well enough. The same can be said for you. If your girlfriend places her trust in you when you go out with your friends, don't act in a way that would betray that trust. Don't make a blunder that could effectively ruin your relationship! That's all there is to it.

LOVE AND IMPROVE YOURSELF

Before a man can learn to love another person, he must first learn to love himself. What you don't have, you can't give. The way you treat yourself is a good indicator of how well you can look after someone else. It's not nearly as difficult as it appears. Make sure you always look out for yourself and you are constantly working on improving yourself. Take care of yourself and exercise regularly. Do what you want, eat what you want, study what you want, and set and achieve your goals! Prioritize the enhancement of your own life above every other thing. The more you develop yourself, the better you'll be able to fulfill your duty as a partner, and the more you improve yourself, the more your spouse will see you as an inspiration to grow as well.

BE A SOURCE OF SAFETY

Your partner must feel safe anytime they are with you for you to be a better man. Your presence must provide a secure environment in which they can let go of their inhibitions and relax. This does not simply imply you should be prepared to defend them if danger arises. It implies you should treat them with discretion. You should be prepared to defend your spouse from anyone attempting to assault them, just as much as you should never do so. Make yourself the safest haven for your partner. It's the very least you can do for them, as a man.

HAVE A SENSE OF HUMOR

A man with a good sense of humor is adored by all. You're well on your way to being a better companion if you can make your partner smile and forget about their difficulties or if you can bring happiness and laughter into a dreary situation. All couples will inevitably experience challenges and misfortunes; it is an integral component of every human relationship. Being someone who offers joy in even the most challenging of circumstances helps ensure the relationship remains strong.

Having said all of that, we are hopeful every young man today challenges themselves to be better and do better for the people they care about. It should be understood relationship maintenance is a continuous process. You continue to tinker at it and refine it and try to make the relationship a better experience for both yourself and your partner. It may seem like a lot to do just to please other people, but if these people in your life are genuine people who love you just as much as you love them, you will find they will start to reciprocate your gestures as well and put in efforts on their end too toward making the relationship work.

Finally, you don't have to be a billionaire, model, or genius to become a better partner. Every man already possesses the necessary building block: character. Your character is what determines your disposition toward making your relationships with other people work. Refine your character by following the tips above to become a better man in your relationships. It's not necessarily the individual things you bring to a relationship; it is the combination of everything. While you might be lacking in one aspect, you can always make up for it by putting in effort and developing your relationship.

CHAPTER 3

MENTAL WHOLENESS

———

International Men's Day is observed on November 19th and is a worldwide celebration of the valuable contributions men make to their communities, families, and the world. This occasion naturally brings up the topic of men's mental health and well-being, which is often disregarded. It may be true a lot of issues relating to mental health are similar in both men and women, but there are some very distinct ones that have been documented to take more of a toll on men. It is therefore important men should begin to prioritize their mental health by engaging in activities that ensure they always operate in a state of mental wholeness.

SO WHAT EXACTLY IS MENTAL WHOLENESS?

In our culture, the term "wholeness" has a variety of meanings. New Age gurus talk about it, preachers preach about it, and pop psychologists talk about it. None of these people, however, can provide a clear definition of what wholeness is. Mental wholeness is even hazier. Many people refer to it, yet no one knows what it means. This could be because the term's meaning is difficult to express, the individual doesn't fully understand what it means, or they simply enjoy the intriguing way it sounds!

Mental completeness is a state of being in which our physical, spiritual, and mental selves are all totally integrated and equal, with none of them dominating the others. Through development and progress, mental wholeness reassembles the damaged pieces of our life—maybe in unexpected ways. Mental wholeness, like physical and spiritual wholeness, is never totally achieved because life is fluid and each day brings new problems. But, like life, completeness is a journey, and we continue to walk it one day at a time.

Above all, mental wholeness is a process that takes a lifetime to complete. It's not something we get quickly, like pain alleviation or learning to handle mental illness through therapy. It's a state we strive toward on a daily basis as we navigate life's ups and downs. Will we be able to tell when we're getting close to anything like wholeness? I'm confident we won't because wholeness breeds humility; the closer we get to wholeness, the more we realize how far we still have to go to achieve balance and integration. Self-care is an important building block for wholeness and should be considered along with these other factors.

IT IS IMPORTANT MEN LEARN TO FOCUS ON THEMSELVES AND NOT ON BEING A "MAN."
Society has made man into a "demigod" in such a way a man can barely do a thing without being asked if he isn't a man—"Are you not a man, you should be. . ." or "You should not. . ." There seems to be so many rules out there kept for

men to follow, and in reality, it is exhausting. In trying to be a "man," you lose yourself and your sanity. So if you must stay mentally whole, be yourself.

Try to be aware of your actions in everyday life to see whether you're doing things merely to appear manly, such as attempting to outdo your friends' stories at the bar, initiating fights for no reason, driving fast, drinking excessively, catcalling women, and avoiding anything girly on principle. Most people will agree abandoning social conventions and expectations to be more authentic requires strong character—so give it a shot!

DEAR MALE FOLK, HOW LONG ARE YOU GOING TO BOTTLE IT UP THIS WAY?

You may probably let out a chuckle when I say "talk to someone," but that's it! Yes, I know what's going through your mind, I know you may be thinking it makes you seem weak, but logically speaking, does it really? I see talking to someone as being courageous enough to face your problems. Need I remind you the first step to solving a problem is admitting you have one? And I definitely think talking to someone is a very brave and strong way of saying, "Hey, I want to get through this."

If you're coping with a mental health condition, another health issue, or any other problem that weighs heavily on your mind, it's crucial to find at least one person you can open up to, whether it's your parent, partner, friend, or counselor. If you don't have somebody to talk to or if you wish to speak to someone anonymously, Good Samaritans are available 24 hours a day, 365 days a year by phone.

MEDITATION AND SELF-AFFIRMATION

Perhaps I will never be able to emphasize this enough for you to see how integral it is in your journey to prioritize mental wholeness. I mean, both things work with the mind, a person's mental state. It is a way of constantly telling your mind to "stay whole" and positive. Yes, meditation may take the form of yoga and similar exercises, but the general idea you must have in mind is to focus your thoughts on positivity.

Have you ever seen someone trying to pull out a snack from a dispensing machine that isn't working properly? The person keeps chanting "I can do it . . . I can . . . almost there . . . " Half of the time, they may not even know they are saying this, but they are telling their subconscious they can actually pull that off, and great news, they do! Affirmations and meditations work the same way.

When you constantly tell yourself you are ugly or too fat, you begin to see yourself as that. It works the same way the other way round. Keep reminding yourself you are enough and you can beat the world. And do this as many times as you can.

Are you familiar with the law of attraction? As revealed by Rhonda Bryne in her book *The Secret,* we are favored with a massive attractive force, one that has no equivalent on the planet, and this force comes from our thoughts. We are capable of changing our entire life with this law of attraction. It is tied in with projecting what we need most in life into our mind and making a powerful thought from it to attract it into our life (Bryne 2006). In essence, the universe gives you whatever you want, whatever you attract, and it is only in the state of your mind. So why don't you stay mentally whole through these things and get what you hope to attract?

TRY DECLUTTERING.

Yes, it's the exact meaning as the term you know. I know we are shouldered with a lot of responsibility, and it is almost normal for us to think a lot, but try decluttering. By this I mean do your best not to think about so many things at the same time. Besides, how do you even do it? The mind has its capacity, and once you begin to overload it with clutter, it breaks down. That's why you realize you soon begin to forget things or have constant migraines or health challenges that are detrimental to your well-being in the long run.

How much does overthinking solve anyway? You can't do everything all at once. Life itself is a process, and we must all learn to follow it one step after the other. Again, just because you are not where you hope to be or what you want to be yet, does not in any way mean you will not get there or achieve those things. Slow down and declutter!

Journaling is a great way to declutter emotionally. Most people think about decluttering being something we do during spring cleaning or when we want to clear out our house. It is a physical thing, but decluttering is something you can do for your mental and emotional well-being too.

GAIN SELF-CONTROL.

It is easy to imagine the idea of self-control being focused on keeping yourself from having that extra piece of cake. While this is an appropriate way of looking at self-control, we also need to make sure to have discipline while looking at emotional and mental issues as well. Learning to control your anger and direct it is just as important as choosing to not have an extra serving of dessert.

The truth is we are often highly susceptible to circumstances that may trigger an outburst of rage if not checked. Stress is one such circumstance. In these situations, it is important to pay more attention to stress and anger management.

When you're in control of your anger, it's a natural and healthy emotion to experience. It's natural to feel angry when we're irritated or being treated unfairly, and it can help us stay motivated and discover personal issues. Because rage usually comes with a sudden "burst of energy," which is part of our natural fight or flight mechanism, it can also help us stay safe and protect ourselves in dangerous situations. However, when your anger drives you to behave in a destructive manner, has a detrimental influence on your mental and physical health, or becomes your default emotion when you want to block out your other emotions, that is not good.

If you feel like you have an anger problem, the following treatments are available:

- Talking therapy and counseling
- Anger management programs
- Help for violent and abusive behavior

Yes, it is possible to be a man who is expressive yet has control over his emotions. In fact, this is ideal.

Here are some extra tips for you; the first is to **get better sleep.** I get it, you're working nine-to-five all the days of the week and you always have unfinished work late at night. But I wouldn't neglect my bedtime if I were you. If robots can get overloaded and break down, men can too.

Sleep and mental health are inextricably linked. Getting a good night's sleep on a regular basis might make you feel less exhausted throughout the day, more capable of coping with everyday chores, more confident with strong self-esteem, and less anxious and agitated. Limit your late-night device usage, do some exercise during the day, eat a balanced diet, and make your bedroom a sleep haven to get a normal seven-to-nine hours of sleep each night.

Are you "hanging with the boys" today because you're stressed and want to unwind? It's a perfect relief, I can't disagree. There's nothing more relaxing than spending time with the people you love. But why do you love drugs and alcohol as much?

Many people consume alcohol or use recreational drugs to unwind or have fun, but other people abuse these substances and use them as a coping mechanisms for stress or other adversity (Anthenelli & Grandison). When men are not feeling well, they are more prone to use drugs and alcohol as coping mechanisms than to seek treatment. Some things, such as weekend binge drinking, are so deeply engrained in our culture you may not even realize you're doing it. Try to be more critical of your alcohol and drug usage to see if you're simply having a good time or if you're burying health problems that would be much better addressed if you admitted them. These things can reduce stress, but when taken in excess, they end up causing more stress and hardship. Never forget substance use affects your mental health.

The importance of mental wholeness cannot be overemphasized. As a man, you should take great care to ensure your mental state is always in the right place. This will ensure better all-round performance in all aspects of your life, as well as an enhanced sense of general well-being. As you can see, there are a ton of issues that go into mental wholeness. Focusing on one of these issues above all others can really unbalance your life and throw everything into chaos. I am proposing a holistic and all-encompassing mind-set that views these issues from above. Like a puzzle, all of these pieces come together to give you the bigger picture.

CHAPTER 4

DEALING WITH TRAUMA

———

The Spirit of the Lord is upon me, because he hath anointed me to preach the gospel to the poor; he hath sent me to heal the brokenhearted, to preach deliverance to the captives, and recovering of sight to the blind, to set at liberty them that are bruised . . .

—LUKE 4.18

We started this book by establishing the importance of self-care of mental health for men. We highlighted the importance of recreational activities and integral self-care activities to keep a man refreshed and energized. And we also looked at the downsides of neglecting mental health care.

This time, we will be taking things a bit deeper. The mind is subdivided into various layers, almost like a complicated maze or a Rubik's cube. It's an advanced biological machine coupled with nuts and bolts sustaining a balanced layer of reality. Men can be subject to trauma too. Our masculinity doesn't shield us from the harsh realities of traumatic events. The issue of trauma in men has not been given the right amount of attention it deserves. It seems as though people don't talk about the subject until something tragic happens such as a mass shooting and the effect can have grand implication. We shall unravel the meaning of trauma and its causes. We are going to look at its unique influence on men and how we can better manage its effects.

AN EXPOSÉ ON TRAUMA

Trauma is the effect of a very unpleasant or tragic events. These events can be so overwhelming they disrupt a person's ability to think properly. Victims of trauma are often left with a feeling of helplessness. Their self-esteem and self-worth take a massive hit and come crashing down like a pack of cards. It's a combination of negative emotions: rage, self-pity, sadness, and depression.

Men are more likely than women to suffer from combat trauma, physical assaults (connected to violent crime) and to witness violence. Similarly, men are more prone than women to get PTSD as a result of combat trauma or rape. Although women are still more likely to be sexually abused as children, it is believed 8 to 29 percent of men were sexually abused as children. It's common for people to view men as intergalactic powerful beings clad in an impenetrable armor of masculinity. Some of us male folks also fancy ourselves to be some type of modern-day Hercules. A fun fact about trauma is it's not scared of our monstrous-looking muscles or rock-solid abs. Physical trauma can be easily diagnosed and treated, but it gets tricky with trauma of the mind.

Several events can cause trauma. It could be anything from the death of a loved one to rape or even natural disasters (hurricanes, earthquakes, that kind of stuff). The reality of this is trauma is not pretty. It's devastating; no one ever wishes to experience a traumatic situation. Trauma affects both men and women, and it deals with everyone the same way, irrespective of race and skin color. According to the World Health Organization's World Mental Health Survey, at least a third of the more than 125,000 adults surveyed in twenty-six nations had experienced trauma. When the group was confined to persons with core disorders, the percentage increased to 70 percent (Pubmed.gov, 2017).

While there are no objective criteria for determining which events may result in post-traumatic symptoms, they usually involve a loss of control, betrayal, power abuse, helplessness, suffering, or disorientation. Such events can cause traumatic effects need not be war, natural disaster, or personal assault. The reality is people react to potentially traumatic events differently. To a large extent, I think it's safe to say it's subjective.

A person who has experienced trauma might react in a variety of ways. They could be in a state of shock, experience deep grief, or denial. Trauma can also cause a variety of long-term effects, including emotional liability, flashbacks, impulsiveness, and damaged relationships. In addition to these, trauma survivors often are extremely sensitive and highly irritable. Trauma can cause physical symptoms such as headaches, fatigue, and nausea, in addition to psychological ones. Some people may be more affected than others. Such individuals may find themselves imprisoned by the traumatic event and find it difficult to go on with their life.

TYPES OF TRAUMA.

Trauma is broadly classified into the distinct categories: Acute, Chronic and Complex Trauma.

ACUTE TRAUMA

Acute Trauma usually occurs as a result of a single traumatic incident, such as an accident, rape, assault, or natural disaster. The situation is serious enough to put the person's mental or physical safety in jeopardy. The event leaves an indelible mark on the individual's psyche. It affects how a person thinks and behaves. This kind of trauma demands immediate medical treatment and therapy. Acute trauma can manifest itself in a variety of ways, including the following:

- Excessive anxiety or panic
- Irritation
- Confusion
- Inability to have a restful sleep
- The feeling of disconnection from your environment
- Unreasonable lack of trust
- Inability to focus on work or studies
- Lack of self-care or grooming
- Aggressive behavior

CHRONIC TRAUMA

This type of trauma occurs when a person is subjected to a series of stressful, long-term, and/or sustained traumatic events. Many men suffer sexual abuse as young boys and tell no one while others endure being bullied in school. In some cases, people suffer the traumatic experiences of war and its horrors, and there seems to be no escape from the sound of rapid gunshots and the picture of lifeless faces. They remember the pain of tragically losing a loved one, and the wounds become fresh all over again. The pain they feel is unbearable and suffocating.

Chronic trauma can also spring from domestic violence. Some grew up under abusive parents who abused them both physically and verbally.

A compilation of acute trauma when it remains untreated can also lead to chronic trauma. Chronic trauma symptoms can take a long time to manifest, even years after the traumatic event occurred. Symptoms include impulsiveness or unpredictable emotional outbursts, anxiety, intense rage, flashbacks, weariness, body aches, headaches, and nausea, among others. Chronic trauma victims may have trust issues, making it difficult for them to maintain secure relationships or work. To recover from the distressing symptoms, such persons would need the assistance of a skilled psychologist (Lifelens).

COMPLEX TRAUMA

Complex trauma is usually the result of being exposed to a variety of negative events or situations. The incidents usually take place in an interpersonal context (between people). This trauma can make a person feel stagnated and grounded. Just like the other types of trauma, complex trauma affects the mind, forming negative and retrogressive mind-sets. Men who have experienced childhood abuse, neglect, marital violence, family disputes, or other recurring events may exhibit complex trauma. It has an impact on a person's overall health, relationships, work, or academic performance (Ibid).

Regardless of what sort of trauma a person suffers, all hope is not lost. If a person is having trouble recovering from their traumatic experiences, they should get professional counseling as soon as possible. A skilled therapist can assist a person who has had a traumatic experience in leading a happy life.

TRAUMA IN MEN
Male Alexithymia: Medical News Today defines Alexithymia as a term used to describe the socialization-induced inhibition of emotional expression in men (Leonard 2019). This is a result of emotional suppression.

Emotions are given to us by God, and they help us better relate with others. As men, we shouldn't suppress our emotion but find a way to positively manage them. Due to some wrong social stereotype, men have been told to suppress their emotions by family members, peers, teachers, coaches, and other role models. Studies have found men with alexithymia might find it challenging to process emotional responses that should naturally follow a traumatic event. So when these men experience traumatic situations, instead of feeling depressed and worried, they become hyper and erratic. Emotional suppression also affects their ability to empathize with people in pain. This is because they have bottled up their emotions to the extent they can't relate to the way others feel. Men suffering from male alexithymia would most likely suck at relationship commitment or even intimacy. "No, no, I hate public displays of affection," he'll say. "Why do we need to take strolls hand in hand like kids?"

The number of men suffering from alexithymia is high, and this only goes to show how twisted the rigid cast of societal dictates could be. But this is a book on healing, so if you're suffering from this, you're in luck. Your emotions are not nonexistent; they are still there, only you've been trained to ignore them. You've been told they make you weak, but they feed you a lie. We are strongest when we feel, when we can connect to the pain of others and see the world through their eyes. Reconnecting to your emotions will be a process. It's going to involve psychotherapy and group therapy. It might start slow at the beginning, but your consistency will yield fruits, best believe that. It's time to connect with family, friends, and the world around you.

AGENTS OF TRAUMA

Typically anything and anyone can be an agent of trauma, but men are more likely to be hurt by strangers or rivals (for example, in combat trauma). Research shows most cases of sexual abuse trauma occur by an abuser within family circles. Men who experienced sexual abuse from someone they know (most commonly in childhood sexual abuse) often grow up to have trust issues arise (US Center of Substance Abuse Treatment). There are general effects of trauma, but most of the time, people respond differently. The following are some notable effects of trauma and their solutions:

- Self-perception: Self-perception is simply the image a person has about themselves. Traumatic events tend to cause a depletion in self-perception. You begin to doubt your abilities, and this can reduce personal development. Thoughts are the instruments of perception, so when a man begins to mentally downgrade himself, then his mind is under the influence of negative thoughts. Negative thoughts can be hard to get away from. They often stic in your mind, and Sometimes, the more you focus on these negative thoughts, the stronger they get. Therefore, it is important to develop ways to distract yourself from them. Many distraction techniques may be helpful, such as deep breathing, self-soothing, and reciting affirmations. Distraction is not about avoidance. Using distraction won't necessarily make those thoughts stop or go away. Distraction may help you, however, take a step back from them, slow them down, or reduce their intensity, making them easier for you to address.

You can further counter those negative thoughts by using positive self-supportive statements. For example, you can list all of your good qualities, tell yourself about what you have accomplished recently that you are proud of, or tell yourself it is okay to feel anxious. You can also list things you are looking forward to in the next week and ask yourself what are some positive ways you have changed recently (either through treatment or just on your own). Lastly, describe a time when you handled your PTSD symptoms well and tell yourself your feelings are valid and important.

HIDDEN FEARS:
Everyone is afraid of something, no matter how to put together they look on the outside. The truth is a little bit of

fear is normal. In fact, fear helps you instinctively protect yourself from harm. Your fear might help you to recognize when you're about to do something dangerous, and it could help you to make a safer choice.

It might be difficult for boys and men to express fear because they have been conditioned to believe men are supposed to be strong and fearless. People could be afraid of other persons, but their greatest foe is themselves and their reactions (acting out after a triggering or upsetting event). This bottled-up fear would soon explode, and boy, the carnage wouldn't be pretty. While fear is simple to conceal in the short term, it can eventually cause problems in long-term relationships. Common ways of facing your fears are evaluating the risks, creating an action plan, seeing a therapist, and being sure not to completely avoid your fears.

The rules are not different for men. Ignoring fears linked to past trauma wouldn't make them magically go away. We must learn to face our fears squarely. Make a sincere estimation of it and you'll realize it's not all that scary. Sometimes, our mind has a way of amplifying things beyond proportion. And even if it's scary as hell, remember in you lies the potential to overcome every setback. Don't let your fears define you, put them in their place! When you do this repeatedly, you'll begin to experience liberty and confidence even as you move past the trauma.

POOR COMMUNICATIVE SKILLS:
Due to gender role norms, men may have more difficulty expressing their trauma. Simply said, being a "victim" does

not fit into the societal stereotype of being a strong man. You're expected to be strong, in control, and able to protect yourself and others. Men feel embarrassed and uncomfortable talking about trauma.

INTIMACY AND SEXUAL ISSUES:

The way men interpret messages about sex and male sexuality from our culture already poses several problems. Sexual assault can further hinder the ability to have a healthy romantic relationship in the future. It's also been proven people who were victims of sexual assaults become sexual predators in the future. Men who have been sexually abused might confuse sex with intimacy, and having relationships with an emotional connection may be a challenge for them.

MEN MAY IGNORE POWER IMBALANCES IN CHILDHOOD SEXUAL ABUSE:

It's not uncommon for boys to have been sexually assaulted by a powerful male figure in their lives, and if this has happened, they would want to keep the abuse a secret and feel deeply embarrassed about the sad event. Some men who have survived sexual assault as adults feel shame or self-doubt, believing they should have been "strong enough" to fight off the perpetrator. Many men who experienced an erection or ejaculation during the assault may be confused and wonder what this means. These normal physiological responses do not in any way imply you wanted, invited, or enjoyed the assault. If something happened to you, know it was not your fault, and you are not alone.

On the other hand, boys who are sexually abused by an older female may perceive the experience as "positive" at first because they have been conditioned to believe any sexual interaction with a female is a good thing. Later on, they may be perplexed by these events and have difficulties classifying them as traumatic or abusive. Sometimes males do not realize the consequences of their experiences until later on when they have children of their own. Overall, the secrecy that comes with traumatic events (especially those related to sexual abuse) prolongs the effects of trauma in its victims.

ANGER:

There is a connecting line between anger and trauma. One way of thinking is high levels of anger are related to a natural survival instinct. When faced with extreme threat, people often respond with anger. Anger can help a person survive by shifting their focus. The person focuses all of their attention, thought, and action toward survival. Anger is also a common response to events that seem unfair or in which you have been made a victim. Research shows anger can be especially common if you have been betrayed by others. This may be most often seen in cases of trauma that involve exploitation or violence. The trauma and shock of early childhood abuse often affects how well the survivor learns to control their emotions. Problems in this area lead to frequent outbursts of extreme emotions, including anger and rage (National Center for PTSD).

In some cases, gender indoctrination encourages males to show anger; it is typically the easiest emotion for them to express (anger equals strength, power, ability to assert oneself). Anger is frequently used as a cover for other feelings males struggle to express, such as grief, frustration, fear, and worry. Their outbursts of rage can be explosive or abusive, and they may use them to push people close to them away. I have met people who are scared of how angry they get over little things.

Their actions often leave them dumbfounded, and they know they need help. Men who are recovering from a traumatic event may require assistance in identifying the emotions behind their anger, as well as learning how to express their anger healthily. But the greatest revelation of strength is in restraint. Being angry with the world can be a bit satisfying; at least, people get to see the effect of the pain you feel. I would recommend acting out in anger to every trauma victim if it heals the heart, but it doesn't.

After serving everyone around you with a dose of rage, you'll redirect it to yourself, and what will be left is self-destruction. So get the help you need today, speak up, and don't die in silence.

TOXIC MASCULINITY & TRAUMA IN MEN

Toxic masculinity is a term used to describe undesirable and typically traditional male qualities or characteristics. Men are frequently defined by obsolete and baseless stereotypes that produce an unhealthy and unrealistic idea of what it means to be a male in today's culture, ranging from being unemotional and power-hungry to narcissistic and violent. Associating men with anger, selfishness, and aggression or assuming men should be guardians, breadwinners, or leaders can cause a lot of trouble. Boys and men are trained to wrongly believe or try to attain lofty and superficial ideas that are based on unproven biases promoted by our society.

Men are significantly more likely than women to commit suicide. Though males are frequently the perpetrators of sexual assault, we often overlook the fact millions of men in our country have also been victims. Male violence, like male victimization, is a problem. According to statistics from the National Sexual Violence Research Center, 5 to 10 percent of girls are victims of penetrative sexual abuse, while 5 percent of guys are also victims of penetrative sexual abuse, which is rarely mentioned. When men and women are charged with the same offense, men are more likely to receive longer terms, with women having a two-to-one advantage in avoiding incarceration.

Anxiety, despair, and mental disease affect both men and women. Men, on the other hand, are more prone than women to underutilize mental health services and be hesitant to seek help, particularly when it comes to mental health. Also, men who purposefully avoid vulnerability, act on homophobic ideas, neglect personal traumas, or engage in discriminatory behaviors toward women contribute to several wider societal issues, including gender-based violence, sexual assault, and gun violence.

Men are typically pressured by society to "be men" in the traditional sense rather than to just be human. Vulnerability is frequently ignored, rejected, or combated by men. Men's mental health suffers when they suppress emotions, neglect sentiments, or dismiss feminine characteristics. We often fail to address the multiple traumas boys and men endure, and we frequently punish actions without addressing the underlying causes that lead to those behaviors. We must remove the stigma associated with mental illness and remind males getting help, expressing emotions, and seeking therapy is not only good but also important for the advancement of our society.

WHAT OUR LADIES CAN DO TO HELP

Goal-oriented and task-oriented therapies may be more effective with men. Always look out for the needs of the men in your life. Take note of specific tasks (e.g., "Let's figure out a time or plan when you/we can go to the gym, go to therapy, see friends, or have more relaxing activities together"). Try to be more supportive than pressuring them to express themselves emotionally if they are not ready. Couples should jot down the emotional signals of their male partner. Men confess to finding it easier to write about their feelings than talk about them.

Trauma is something that can and will affect men across the board. We need to be aware of the different types of trauma and the effects they can have on men. Once we are able to identify and analyze these traumas, we are better able to deal with them and use them to further our own sense of self, making us better men in the long run.

CHAPTER 5

THE AWAKENING: HEALING THROUGH SELF-EXAMINATION

One of the main opportunities to come from trauma is the ability to heal, making yourself a better man in the long run. Learning to improve yourself through self-examination is very important through your life's journey as a man. It is almost ridiculous how society says, "man up" and we as men obediently learn to bottle up every hurt, pain, trauma, and emotion. But the truth is no matter how much effort we put into hiding these feelings, they can never be hidden well enough. No matter how invisible we try to make our emotions, life always tells on it in the most unpredicted ways possible.

Healing suggests some sort of breakthrough from something ill or negative. It is important to know no one grows with pain, fear, or whatever negativity around them—absolutely no one at all. Pain kills motivation to chase dreams even creating stuck points that drain life energy. Thus, as an evolving man, you can only become better off when you allow yourself to heal.

Health wise, nothing is as sought after as healing is. Whether it is from an illness, an injury, a surgery etc. It is probably why doctors would suggest you "take a rest" during and after treatment. It's like a way of saying "allow yourself to heal." Look at it this way: literally no one loves to stare at an open wound forever. It reminds us the pain is still there, we're still hurt, and this is not a great feeling at all. It is difficult to get on with our lives when we are not fully healed. It's the reason why a person who broke their wrists cannot carry things or write until after a certain period of time when healing has taken place fully. So it is safe to say such conditions or injuries may pose a limitation in our lives.

To put this in real sense: nothing ever works when we do not heal. It is hard to deal with looming pain, and even worse, when we're in pain, we can never get a hold of our lives. For instance, take a child who just lost his parents, a husband with a problematic marriage, or even a boy who had experienced a lot of trauma growing up. Throughout their lives, these victims would be constantly affected in one way or another. The orphan could be affected psychologically and have a different ideal about life, and this may or may not be reflected in his relationship with others. The husband could decide never to believe in the institution of marriage, and the little boy may raise his family the same way. This goes to stress the dire importance of healing. If we want to become better people, we ought to look beyond these pains and figure a way to get out of it. Some wounds are impossible to heal from, but in that case, while you may not fully heal, you can use the situation and what you learned to better yourself still.

Fear and anxiety would stop you from reaching a goal in life. I know of a child who always feared getting on a bicycle because he fell off it once. When the little kids his age were cycling down the empty streets, he sat in a corner watching them sorrowfully, only wishing he could join them and not miss out on all the fun they were having. But he couldn't because he feared if he got on a bike, he would fall off and hurt himself again. It is apparent the child in question had an experience he hasn't yet healed from. Needless to say this dilemma he has found himself in has greatly limited him from having fun with his peers (yet he really wants it). But is it really worth it?

I'll draw many more illustrations to other emotions like guilt and shame. Let's say for instance, you did something shameful and wrong many years ago and the guilt of your actions still lurks in your mind. How well do you think you can grow in such an environment? You constantly abuse yourself when you flood your mind with this unhealthy emotion.

I wouldn't leave grief out. Everyone has at one time or another lost someone or something that was really important to them and they held dear to their heart. Extreme cases of grief have changed people's lives forever and have made some resort to more severe cases of self-abuse and self-harm.

WHY IS IT IMPORTANT THAT YOU MUST HEAL?

Yes we are human, and for this, we are permitted to feel all these things as there are no strange feelings; that's no debate. But being in denial about unresolved trauma becomes a problem in the long run because in times like these, we are left unsure of what to do and struggle to get through life. We find ourselves rapidly moving toward negativity, and that affects our emotional, physical, and mental balance and general well-being in a way that is destructive. We may not see it immediately, but these negatives reveal themselves as we go on in life. This is what I implied earlier when I said, "life will tell on it."

Healing is essential. It helps us acknowledge and face our circumstances while learning to create ways to help ourselves become better. Yes, as I have noted, these circumstances are capable of changing our lives forever. This is why it is essential to take our lives by the reins while it is early and move on to healing. There is no better way to heal than through proper self-examination.

SELF-EXAMINATION & HEALING

I would say the most appropriate way to define self-examination is by using the term "reflection." Otherwise, I would rather conceptualize it to be everything aimed at self-improvement through a careful study of one's life, patterns, and behavior. The concept of self-examination can be likened to taking a school test or exams. You've been taught lessons in school, and after a few, you were given a test to see how well you had learned your lessons. When you failed such tests, you went back to look at the areas you did poorly in and study to become better and stronger in those areas, right?

Self-examination works exactly the same way. It's reflecting on your past, the mistakes, challenges, and lessons and seeking ways in which you can use this knowledge to grow and improve your future. In a single phrase, self-examination is "growing from your past."

I know it is quite the trend to say, "let bygones be bygones" or "bury the past in the past," but the sooner we realize the past always haunts our future if we do not handle it well, the better for all of us. I do not say this to mean "brood over your past." No! That is unhealthy and totally unacceptable. What is acceptable is looking back at your life in past times with hope for a better tomorrow. Find silver lining lessons learned from these past events to change the actions in the present so the future is better

The Bible even commands Christians in Romans 12:2:

> "Do not become so well-adjusted to your culture that you fit into it without even thinking. Instead, fix your attention on God. You'll be changed from the inside out. Readily recognize what he wants from you, and quickly respond to it. Unlike the culture around you, always dragging you down to its level of immaturity, God brings the best out of you, develops well-formed maturity in you."

The simple explanation of this Bible verse is: Don't get to used to being what you are now or what you used to be. Always try to be better while looking up to God.

CAN YOU HEAL WHEN YOU DO NOT KNOW WHAT YOU'RE HEALING FROM?

I bet you can answer that for yourself. Self-examination helps you understand there is a problem, as well as helping you identify it. Have you ever gone to the clinic to see the doctor and upon seeing you, they started writing out prescriptions that would help you heal? I'm certain no! This is quite the same; self-examination acts like a medical diagnosis. In its simplicity, it helps you think "Why do I act this way? How does this behavior affect my life? What lessons have I learned from this experience? Are the lessons from the experience negative or positive?" Then, you can offer solutions like "How can I do better?"

Freddie, for instance, is a boy who grew up in one of those homes people love to describe as "hanging on a thin rope." His father was quite abusive, and his mother almost always neglected him. No adult in the home validated Freddie, he wasn't told he was loved. It was indeed a traumatic experience for Freddie, as he never got the chance to feel what it was like to be in a stable, normal home. So Freddie grew up this way. Fast-forward to several years later: The young boy has become a man and has seemed to find the woman he is willing to spend the rest of his life with. But there is one problem.

Ellie, his fiancée doesn't agree with his notion women have to be the punching bags and underdogs in relationships. She is not ready to be in a relationship that would cost her life, and after enduring his excesses for months, she leaves his life.

Of course Freddie was broken and regretful, but it was too late. It is rather difficult to convince a woman or anyone at all domestic violence is "just a mistake that won't happen again." He'd grown up seeing this all the time, so it didn't seem wrong or strange to him until he realized it was. At that time, he remembered all of his childhood and how hard it had been for him. He realized the same trait was now gaining presence and possible dominance in his life, and no, he didn't want that. So a few months after, Freddie chose to become better; he went for therapy, learned self-control, and yes, found love again! I promise it's a "happily ever after" story.

In like ways, reflecting on ourselves, past experiences, and mistakes helps us take informed steps to prevent such mistakes from happening the second time. It gives you the chance to channel your emotions positively for a positive outcome.

HEALING AND SELF-EXAMINATION IN PRACTICE

I want to walk you through a simple exercise to show you what I have been talking about. This is what self-examination looks like in practice. However, areas where you need to examine yourself may differ and questions you need to ask yourself may differ too depending on the context in which you take the exercise. Nevertheless, the procedures are similar:

- Challenge yourself by asking questions
- Give yourself unbiased answers

- Say how these self-examination questions and unbiased answers have affected your life and how you can work with these to become better
- And . . . action!!!

STEP #1: CHALLENGE YOURSELF BY ASKING QUESTIONS

For some people, it is a question of who they really are, their strengths, their weakness, and their general life experiences. Who am I? What's my purpose? What are my strengths? What's my greatest regret? And so on. It is an in-depth account of who they truly are from their own perspective. Ask yourself as many questions as you wish to. It is necessary you do to grasp what you're all about.

Now, the question I'd love to ask you here is . . . *What has your life been like in the past five years?*

STEP #2: GIVE YOURSELF UNBIASED ANSWERS

Pause for a second, think, and do not just rush to answer. The question holds more depth than you're about to make it seem. And it is same for any other question you may decide to ask yourself too.

What has life been like? Tough? Hard to deal with? Blissful? Pressurizing? Indifferent? Full of experiences?

The answer to the question asked in step one should aim at giving a thorough description of your entire journey including your strengths, weaknesses, mistakes, and achievements.

Generally, provide yourself with an answer feasible enough to work with.

STEP #3: SAY HOW THESE HAVE AFFECTED YOUR LIFE AND HOW YOU CAN WORK WITH THESE TO BECOME BETTER

Let's say I answered by saying my life has been full of experiences in the past five years. I may now answer the A part of this step by saying it has made me see life as a journey full of lessons; I've made a lot of mistakes, a lot of which I regret and some I have learned from. And in the B part, I hope to fall back to the lessons I've learned in the future and try to avoid the same mistakes again.

STEP #4: AND . . . ACTION!!!

Wake up and manifest greatness. Be better! This step also entails a lot of self-affirmation and meditation. These two work hand in hand to help instill the confidence you need to be where you want to be. Say words like "I can do this, there's greatness in me, I am enough" because you are. Look into the mirror every day and remind yourself of that thing you want to become, the better man you hope to be. By doing so, you instill greatness in your subconscious. Write it everywhere, say it every time, but yes, it's not enough to just talk; stand up and support your talking with action.

Using an example, I'll put these four steps into practice in one paragraph:

"What's my life been like in the past 5 years? In the past five years, I've been dealing with inconsistency and temperamental issues. I've been affected by these at work, my temperament has made me take unruly decisions and hurt people, and my inconsistency has made me less productive. I'd be a better co-worker if I learned to control my temper and could also be very successful if I stay patient and consistent."

Self-affirmation would look like:

- "I am enough, and I can be great."
- "I have the power to control my feelings."
- "I will not make rash decisions."
- Remember, the last step is to take action, always!

Dear reader, healing is a process. And I must note as such, you can't complete all phases of self-examination and healing in one go. A sore doesn't magically disappear; it heals gradually. However, certain things can be given or taken to hasten the healing process. In the context at hand, only determination and consistency can heal you quickly, but that's not yours to decide, so don't rush it. Let healing take its full course and watch yourself fully evolve into the exquisite man you are. While your journey may differ, hopefully these steps can help guide you along the path!

CHAPTER 6

FINDING PURPOSE

—

"This is the true joy of life: the being used up for a purpose recognized by yourself as a mighty one; being a force of nature instead of a feverish, selfish little clot of ailments and griev-ances, complaining that the world will not devote itself to making you happy."

GEORGE BERNARD SHAW

Purpose is the nebula of life. It is the combustion that fuels and energizes men to have satisfactory existence. The words of Dr. Myles Munroe are everlasting and true when he says; "If the purpose of a thing is unknown, abuse is inevitable." Just how important could purpose be in the grand scheme of things? Is it worth the countless books and articles written on the subject matter? Many might play with this question in their mind because it's easier to live life mindlessly than intentionally.

Now and then, we face the temptation to live life aimlessly, to chill and flow with whatever life throws at us. But I've found out only purpose-driven people are successful. The research on purpose is very impressive. There are health benefits to living purposefully. People with a sense of purpose are less likely to experience a stroke or become addicted to alcohol and drugs. Having a sense of purpose appeared to be more important for decreasing risk of death than drinking, smoking, or exercising regularly, according to a study published in JAMA.

In fact, in a long-term study conducted by Rush University, a group of adults were monitored as the adults aged. The subjects reported their sense of purpose throughout the study. Interestingly, those who reported to having a sense of purpose were twice as likely to be free of the symptoms of cognitive decline, dementia, and Alzheimer's. The scientists studied their brains after they passed away and were surprised by what they found: purpose had protected their brains from displaying the effects of aging, even though some of their brains showed the physical signs of cognitive degeneration.

Finding purpose is more of a journey than a spontaneous inspirational moment. And we've been on that journey all our lives, making stops, hitting bumps, and sometimes falling flat on our faces. Such is the highway of life. One of the greatest dilemmas men face is centered around purpose. You have people around you trying to define what your life should be like. Plus, the society we live in doesn't make it any easier.

Men are almost under constant pressure to be or act in a certain way. If he cries, it would be said he's acting like a baby, he should be more like a man. If he displays his masculinity, some may see that as egoistic. Decades ago, being nice and helpful to a lady was seen as what it is: a human being simply being nice to another human being. But now, chivalry is dead they say. Men have been accused of using chivalry to downplay the abilities of women. I'm trying to get you to see how confusing it is to be a man in this age and time and why the importance of purpose cannot be overestimated.

One of the greatest truths of purpose is it can be deciphered from the design of the object of inquiry. For example, let's take a person with no knowledge of how a chair works seeing a chair and instinctively sitting on it because he's tired. It is the same reason every smartphone creator places a user manual in the products package. To properly understand purpose, we must first understand our unique configuration as men. Men often feel dissatisfied with failure. They are more logical (not necessarily smarter), more driven, hungrier to make a name for themselves. This passion, if not well coordinated, could put a person on the wrong path in life.

There are two extremes when it comes to a man's pursuit of a better life. In the first, he is so pumped and passionate in his pursuit he is willing to ignore values and harm his mental health. This could have a far-reaching effect on a person. In the other extreme, he's laid-back, lazy, and not willing to put in the necessary effort to advancing in life. Finding purpose is the equilibrium between both extremes. A man who knows and lives by his purpose would often overcome laziness and get the job done pronto. Purpose also serves as a guard rail for him, protecting him from harming himself in the process.

WHAT DRIVES YOUR LIFE?

Everyone's life is driven by something. Most dictionaries define the verb drive as "to guide, to control, or to direct." Whether you are driving a car, a nail, or a golf ball, you are guiding, controlling, and directing it at that moment. What is the driving force in your life? Right now, you may be driven by a problem, pressure, or a deadline. You may be driven by a painful memory, a haunting fear, or an unconscious belief. There are hundreds of circumstances, values, and emotions that can drive your life.

Here are two of the most common ones:

Many people are driven by **guilt**. They spend their entire lives running from regrets and hiding their shame. Guilt-driven people are manipulated by memories. They allow their past to control their future. They often unconsciously punish themselves by sabotaging their own success. We are products of our past, but we don't have to be prisoners of it. It doesn't matter what ugly thing your past holds, you can open up a new chapter and start living again.

Many people are driven by resentment and **anger**. They hold on to hurts and never get over them. Instead of releasing their pain through forgiveness, they rehearse it over and over in their minds. Some resentment-driven people "clam up" and internalize their anger, while others "blow up" and explode it onto others.

Both responses are unhealthy and unhelpful. Resentment always hurts you more than it does the person you resent. While your offender has probably forgotten the offense and gone on with life, you continue to stew in your pain, perpetuating the past. Listen: Those who have hurt you in the past cannot continue to hurt you now unless you hold on to the pain through resentment. Your past is past! Nothing will change it. You are only hurting yourself with your bitterness. For your own sake, learn from it, and let it go. The Bible says, "To worry yourself to death with resentment would be a foolish, senseless thing to do," Job 5:2 (GNT). Many people are driven by fear. Their fears may be a result of a traumatic experience, unrealistic expectations, having growing up in a high-control home, or even genetic predisposition. Regardless of the cause, fear-driven people often miss great opportunities because they're afraid to venture out. Instead, they play it safe, avoiding risks and trying to maintain the status quo.

Fear is a self-imposed prison that will keep you from becoming what you've been predestined to be. You must move against it with the weapons of faith and love. Many people are driven by materialism. Their desire to acquire becomes the whole goal of their lives. This drive to always want more is based on the misconceptions having more will make you more happy, more important, and more secure, but all three ideas are untrue. Possessions only provide temporary happiness. Because things do not change, we eventually become bored with them and want newer, bigger, better versions. It's also a myth if I get more, I will be more important. Self-worth and net worth are not the same. Your value is not determined by your valuables, and the most valuable things in life are not things! The most common myth about money is having more will make you more secure. It won't. Wealth can be lost instantly through a variety of uncontrollable factors.

FINDING YOUR PURPOSE

I used to think finding purpose was like the traditional Easter egg hunt, if I checked hard and long enough, I would find it hidden in some mysterious location. I couldn't have been more wrong. Purpose is not something you find in a eureka moment. Finding purpose is not an event but a journey. It's a journey we begin from the very moment we became mindful and conscious of our unique personalities. This is why children ask a lot of questions; they are simply trying to figure out their identity and how to relate with the world around them. The first step to finding your purpose is to first believe you have one in the first place. You were created for something bigger than you. These words are not to make you feel good, it's just what it is!

If you are reading this book, then I'm most certain you want to develop your life beyond its current state. It's like starting life all over again but getting it right this time. You possibly might have lived impulsively before now and fell into a lot of mistakes. But see, we're going to do some exercises to help you heal and discover purpose (or rediscover purpose, for some).

Let's do a bit of introspection, can we? What makes you tic? What's that very thing that constantly echoes in your heart, consciously or subconsciously? I've discovered no man is exactly the same. We may share similarities, but deep within our hearts, we have a unique structure. It's easy to neglect the passions of our hearts because they seem normal; but what if they indeed hold clues to what you are meant to be doing on Earth?

This is time for some honest soul-searching. Successful men in life share an identical trait: They had a burden that weighed heavily on their hearts, a problem they would have given anything to solve, something they would have gladly invested their all into. And guess what, it has always been there. Chances are you have an idea of what it is, but you just have not searched deeper. The deeper you go, the more you know and the more convinced you will be. What I'm trying to say in essence is you are a solution to a present-day problem. You have a unique purpose. You're more than a statistic. You must realize if you don't live out your purpose, people will be the worse for it!

Another indicator of purpose could be ease of operation. Have you ever noticed how certain things just come easily for you without much effort? You could watch with bewilderment how people struggle with those same things, but for you, it's a piece of cake, a walk in the park. A person's purpose and potential works hand in hand. It's safe to say we are given gifts and talents to equip us in advancing our purposes more efficiently. Take a pen and list out those gifts and natural inclinations you have, and you'll be able to draw a purpose map of how you should use them.

My natural gifts, list them here:

BENEFITS OF PURPOSEFUL LIVING

Focus: the ability to set your heart and mind on a goal and follow it through. Focus has to do with the singleness of your gaze. This is one of the products of living with purpose. It helps you direct your energies toward a definite direction, and by doing so, we become more successful. You can set the right order of priorities in your life. It is easier to choose the things that would help you advance on the path you have discovered. It's also easier to do away with needless and counterproductive things. This is very necessary because we live in a world of so many voices and distractions, and it has become increasingly easy to drift away if we lose our focus. It might look intriguing to do a lot of things, but in life, you must narrow in on a selected few if you want to be successful.

Knowing your purpose gives meaning to your life. We were made to have meaning. This is why people try dubious methods, like astrology or psychics, to discover it. When life has meaning, you can deal with almost anything; in its absence, life becomes unbearable. Finding purpose gives you a refreshing sense of faith and hope. I love the following quote from Rick Warren's book, *Purpose Driven Life*. A young man in his twenties wrote, "I feel like a failure because I'm struggling to become something, and I don't even know what it is. All I know how to do is to get by. Someday, if I discover my purpose, I'll feel I'm beginning to live." If you've not found a cause worth dying for, then you've not found a reason life is worth living. But then again, purpose gives our lives definition—isn't that what we're all looking for as men?

Knowing your purpose motivates your life. Purpose always produces passion. Nothing energizes like a clear purpose. On the other hand, passion dissipates when you lack a purpose. Just getting out of bed becomes a major chore. It is usually meaningless work, not overwork, that wears us down, saps our strength, and robs our joy. George Bernard Shaw wrote, "This is the true joy of life: the being used up for a purpose recognized by yourself as a mighty one; being a force of nature instead of a feverish, selfish little clot of ailments and grievances, complaining the world will not devote itself to making you happy."

We don't have eternity on Earth, and if we must reach our full potential as men, we must learn to live purposefully, numbering our days and striving for the difference we've been destined to make.

CHAPTER 7

THE ART OF SELF-MOTIVATION

———

Just like Kung Fu, Tai Chi, or painting a pretty picture on a canvas, self-motivation is an art. Ever been in a mental place where you know what to do but can't find the strength to do it? Then you're left feeling like a failure, an utter disappointment. This is a battle men face in general, but especially those who have been through traumatic life events. When traumatic events collide with the mind, it scatters the hopes and the dreams we had and all that's left is a hollow void that seems impossible to fill. The journey back to mental wholeness is not complete until we master the art of self-motivation. We discussed purpose in the last chapter and its importance to healing and success. Now you know what purpose is and its importance, it's time to find the motivation you need to drive your purpose.

Motivation can be simply described as the force behind your behavior. It's the "why" behind everything you do. Every commitment a person makes to a cause or an action has a driving motivation behind it. Everything we do is motivated by some combination of conscious and unconscious need or desire.

Self-motivation is the art of pushing oneself to take initiative and action to pursue goals and complete tasks. It's an intrinsic drive to take action—to create and to achieve. It's what keeps you moving even when you're out of steam, especially when you're pursuing a task because you want to, not because someone told you to.

The reason why this concept is so important to the well-being of men is we don't achieve our goals in a day. We have long-term goals and short-term goals, and the process of achieving these goals might not always be straightforward. When reaching for a big goal, self-motivation plays a key role. Say you're trying to right the wrongs in your life and you passionately want things to be different this time. If you want to quit a harmful habit, get healthy, make a midlife career change, or realize a personal dream, you'll notice the beginning is always easy. You're full of enthusiasm and determination to face any challenge, but one thing we often fail to factor in is most of our goals don't happen quickly. It's going to take hard work, persistence, and discipline to change your life. When your desired result is stalling and it seems like nothing is going right, it's natural to feel frustrated and have difficulty staying motivated.

Self-motivation here transcends basic motives. What we really mean is the ability to follow through on making a positive change in life without throwing in the towel. Self-motivation requires you believe in your potential and abilities.

You must build confidence and draw inspiration even in the face of setbacks.

Psychologist Angela Duckworth studied the characteristics of high achievers and discovered passion and perseverance are the key drivers of long-term success. Grit takes you farther than the initial motive behind your goal after the buzz of excitement wears off. Grit takes you to the finish line. An interesting explanation comes to mind that will better describe the concept of grit (Duckworth, 2016). Your mind responds in the way you train it to respond. You might say to yourself, "Train my mind? I don't remember doing that," but you sure have. The way you respond to circumstances trains the mind to respond to future experiences in the same way.

The training of the mind can either be conscious or unconscious. My goal for you is you get to a place where you can consciously train your mind to think and respond to situations positively. This is key to sustaining a healthy mental environment. The mind is a muscle. Muscles can tear, they can heal, and most importantly, they can be trained to be tough and strong. This is basically how **grit works**.

SELF-MOTIVATION THEORY

Psychologists have contributed by proposing theories to try to explain why we are motivated to do (or not to do) different things. For example, Maslow's hierarchy of needs theory suggests we are innately driven to meet important psychological needs like belonging and self-esteem. Self-determination theory suggests individuals have different levels of motivation based on how intrinsically or extrinsically motivated we are.

This theory also suggests universal needs such as competence, autonomy, and relatedness motivate our behavior.

THE RELATIONSHIP BETWEEN DEPRESSION AND MOTIVATION

"A merry heart doeth good like a medicine: but a broken spirit drieth the bones"

PROV.17.22

This is one of the chief enemies of self-motivation. Depression attacks your desire to step out and get things done. It can be experienced at different levels; it may seem like all you can do is watch TV or lie in bed, but extreme cases are characterized by suicidal thoughts. Feeling low and unmotivated makes it even harder to recover from trauma or other forms of mental disorders.

If you are experiencing low moods and feeling more and more tired, you're not alone. Feeling down, even for basic self-care, has been linked to an imbalance of the brain chemicals that are responsible for emotion and behavior. Motivation is the result of a complex network of chemical and electrical signals in the brain. Things can and will go south with both mood and motivation when these chemicals are imbalanced.

While the major cause of depression to most people is inadequate amounts of serotonin, there are many other chemical factors involved in the onset of depression. These chemicals, called neurotransmitters, are responsible for signaling different nerves or brain cells. They are chemical messengers with distinct messages that could cause depressive symptoms if they fail to deliver. There are many different types of neurotransmitters, and they all have cooperative and overlapping functions. Neurotransmitters control actions in our minds and bodies, including but not limited to:

- Focus/alertness
- Sleep
- Motor behavior/movements
- Addiction/reward
- Muscle function
- Mood
- Memory and learning
- Some neurotransmitters speed up signals while others slow down brain synapses. When some move too fast and others not fast enough, they contribute to depression and anxiety.

THE BIOLOGY OF DEPRESSION

In addition to serotonin imbalances, disrupted dopamine signaling has been shown to affect depression, especially feelings of excitement and motivation. When the mind experiences intense stress, it might temporarily increase dopamine levels followed by a reduction. These decreases in dopamine are an explanation behind the emptiness we feel after experiencing an intensely stressful situation. According to an NIH study involving rats, those who exhibited traits of helplessness and lacked the motivation to escape a negative foot shock stimulus had a 50 percent reduction in dopamine firing. If depression is preventing you from living your fullest life, dopamine regulation may represent a valuable target in your treatment plan.

WHY DO PEOPLE BURN OUT?

Burnout is another enemy of self-motivation. When you come under intense pressure, your natural survival response kicks in, causing cortisol (a stress hormone) to rise. Most men face similar stressors like jobs, finances, family, relationships, commuting, and so on. Prolonged stress can make impactful changes to our body's natural cortisol rhythm. When your cortisol rhythm shifts, your body produces varying levels of cortisol at different times, and the effect is it leaves you exhausted to complete your daily tasks. There is a clear link between burnout, depression, and lack of motivation, and it is important to consider the impact of chronic stress on mental health.

THE SOLUTION

I hope you weren't bored with all the science talk. We must understand the science sponsoring the enemies of our motivation if we hope to overcome them. Fortunately, there are many ways you can put this knowledge into action. You've done the first part in informing yourself about the science of mental health and neurotransmitters.

Recent research reveals inflammation, which is an important factor in the development of depression, can reduce dopamine signaling in the brain, and living and maintaining a healthy lifestyle can work wonders for you. Eating well, getting enough sleep, and incorporating movement into your daily routine are excellent ways to decrease inflammation. If you find yourself less motivated and your mood has declined significantly, you will want to look into seeking a diagnosis, treatment, and management for depression.

Beyond all these, the best remedy to heal a depressed heart is crying out to God just like King David did.

"Why, my soul, are you downcast? Why so disturbed within me? Put your hope in God, for I will yet praise him, my Savior and my God."

PSALM 42:11

There is nothing you might be going through God can't help you sort out. If you're feeling overwhelmed, take a piece of paper and write down all the blessings your higher power showers on you daily, and fresh strength will flow into your heart.

WHAT DRIVES MOTIVATION?

Although self-motivation is a journey, it's important to look at what is motivating you to seek change. The clearer you are on the "why," the easier it will be to remain focused on the work and your life's purpose and create the life you want.

Sometimes our motives might hide in plain sight, buried in our subconscious, telling us deep down something needs to change. Our desires evolve, sometimes in a flash of inspiration, and in other times through self-discovery. I speak from experience when I say it's easier to stay motivated when we recognize the motives behind our goals. Becoming aware of these motives and where they originate from improves self-awareness while also keeping you on track as you pursue your goals. According to Deci Edward, author of *Intrinsic Motivation*, the nature of your motivation can be described in two ways. They include **intrinsic and extrinsic motivation** (Deci 1975, 129).

Intrinsic motivation describes when your drive is powered by **internal factors**. Intrinsically motivated men are motivated not because of external rewards, like money or recognition, but a sense of personal reward. This is quite rare, something the average man might struggle with. It's easier to gain motivation from an external source than to build an internal motivational structure and reward system. When we pull through and do the things we didn't feel like doing, we experience a fresh release of strength and confidence. Part of being self-motivated is having good levels of self-assurance, self-confidence, and self-efficacy. More on these below!

Being highly self-assured means you will set challenging goals for yourself, and it's also a resiliency factor for when you encounter setbacks. If you don't believe in yourself, you'll be much more likely to think, "I knew I couldn't do this" instead of, "This one failure isn't going to stop me!"

Albert Bandura, a psychologist from Stanford University, defined self-efficacy as a belief in our own ability to succeed and our ability to achieve the goals we set for ourselves. This belief has a huge impact on your approach to goal setting and your behavioral choices as you work toward those goals. In other words, our deepest desires, wants, and dreams come from within and drive self-motivation. Some examples of intrinsic motivation include:

- changing habits to feel healthier,
- pursuing a lifelong dream, or
- building stronger and more meaningful relationships with people.

What heartfelt desires drive you to become a better person and pursue your dreams? That's where you will find intrinsic motivation.

Extrinsic motivation refers to being driven by external rewards. Men wired this way often aim to attain some kind of reward, such as money, status, or good performance. Examples include studying hard in the quest for perfect grades in school, hitting sales goals at work, or changing the way you look to win people's approval.

Everyone is different. We all come from different backgrounds and upbringings, therefore, each person has their own set of intrinsic or extrinsic motivations. Whether you feel more encouraged by internal motivation or find yourself influenced by the external or both, neither is right or wrong. The important thing is you find the balance between being intrinsically and extrinsically motivated. Although both aren't wrong, you want to make sure to recognize motivators so you can avoid chasing empty goals. Motivation is good, but it's more rewarding and satisfying to be motivated by the right reasons.

Self-motivation is one trait employers look for when selecting new staff into their workforce. A self-motivated employee will:

- Start tasks promptly and finish them on time
- Initiate new projects that can benefit the business
- Stay focused on work and put off every distraction.

A self-motivated roommate will:

- Make sure to clean the house when it gets messy
- Keep the grass cut
- Never leave dirty plates in the sink

A self-motivated husband or fiancéeé will;

- Be kind and loving to his partner
- Shower her frequently with words of affirmation.
- Work through problems instead of running away

Here are some examples of traits that self-motivated men have:

- **Drive to achieve.** The desire to accomplish something versus working for external rewards like money or prestige.
- **Initiative.** The tendency to act, take charge, or move forward before others do.
- **Resilience.** The ability to keep going despite difficulties.
- **Commitment to goals.** The persistence to reach goals.
- **Passion for work.** The enjoyment of the work itself.
- **Desire to improve.** The need to keep getting better (Goleman, 2017).

- **Eagerness.** The desire to try new things and take on new challenges.
- **Self-efficacy.** The belief that your actions will lead to desired results (Stajkovic & Luthans, 1998).

TIPS TO FIND MOTIVATION

Getting back to a good mental space of self-motivation is not easy. There will be days when you think you have things going your way only to have them crumble. Finding self-motivation requires long-term commitment, courage, and perseverance. But that doesn't mean it's impossible. It simply means you have to find ways to give yourself a boost when you need it and avoid giving up when you hit a dip.

I'll be proposing helpful tips to stay motivated, no matter how much you feel like giving up:

1. FOCUS YOUR ENERGY

A life of simplicity creates an enabling environment for self-motivation. It will keep distractions at bay and prevent you from feeling overwhelmed, especially during times of disruption. Simplicity creates room in our heads and hearts to become creative and grow despite the challenges we face. There is a verse in the Bible that explains this perfectly:

Therefore I do not run like someone running aimlessly; I do not fight like a boxer beating the air.

1 COR 9:26

A person who lacks focus would be all over the place. Note activity is not necessarily productivity. Instead of trying to do so many things at once, choose your area of focus. This will not only help simplify your life but will enable you to direct all your talents toward your most important goal. Aim to become badass in one area instead of halfheartedly working in many areas at once.

2. BREAK DOWN LARGE GOALS INTO SMALL STEPS

The journey of a thousand miles begins in a day, they say. Estimate the larger goal and consider the small steps to achieve it. Break things down into digestible bits and work on them. This will help you celebrate your wins as you hit your targets. This is a common habit in successful people, and it works well to make large goals more attainable.

3. MANAGE YOUR EXPECTATIONS

You've put a great deal of work into a project, be it a personal or professional project. But you don't see progress as quickly as you expect, or your plans sort of hit a snag. At this point, frustration can set in, and you may be tempted to give up. As obstacles pile up, frustration becomes despair, and you may tell yourself, "This goal is not attainable."

Your brain is constantly calculating whether or not it's worth the effort to keep going. In the book Burnout, authors Emily Nagoski, PhD, and Amelia Nagoski, DMA, call this concept "The Monitor"(Nagoski, 2019). It's the process in your brain that keeps a running tally of the effort-to-progress ratio in any undertaking. The monitor of the mind often sets unrealistic goals. If you get entangled with the emotions attached to failure, you'll never rise to the top. No matter how many times you've failed, you can achieve your goals.

There is always a night of the soul, and your nerves may weaken. You should expect a dip in which momentum slows down or the trajectory seems wobbly. Your job in staying motivated is to find ways to manage the stress and emotional turmoil of the inevitable dips and keep going. You have to believe in yourself and your capabilities (Soulsault, 2021).

4. SURROUND YOURSELF WITH SUPPORTIVE PEOPLE

As iron sharpens iron, so a friend sharpens a friend.

- PROV.27.17

The people around you matter. Whatever you call them homies, brothers, or friends, you must have them around you, and not just any friend—the right type of friend, friends who help us stay in touch with our desired outcomes. People who have a significant support system or even one supportive person in their corner fare better than those going at it alone.

The weight of life's issues weighs us down if we don't have effective human support systems. These are people who can see our mess and still lovingly push us to do better and stay positive.

In her best-selling book, Conversational Intelligence, Judith E. Glaser explains how supportive people can step in to guide and motivate us like a coach during a football game. During the game of life in which we pursue our goals, positive people can help you reframe, redirect, and refocus when it gets tough (Glaser, 2016). On the other hand, the wrong people and the wrong environment could cause psychological and physical distress that derail progress toward positive goals.

5. LEARN TO ASK FOR HELP

One classic trait of men is an unreasonable phobia of asking for help. Some think it makes them look weak or less masculine, but this is a misguided perspective. When you're trying to stay motivated in your quest, the right help can be the difference between success and giving up. According to Professor Richard Boyatzis who has studied motivation for decades, we can all benefit from becoming better at offering and receiving the right kind of coaching (Harvard Business Review, 2019).

Beyond asking for help, we must practice offering help also. The rivers of our charity and benevolence must flow freely. It's common for most folks to offer help in a mode called "coaching for compliance." This is when you're trying to fix someone or get them to do what you want. Even if the advice is sound, this approach does not work to create lasting positive change. The person on the receiving end can sniff it the moment you begin. They'll feel like you're imposing it upon them, making learning and growth difficult.

The most effective approach is called "coaching with compassion." This coaching style is not about helping but about caring. Conversations with great coaches tie your goals back to your values and dreams. By adding context, they boost self-motivation and openness to new ideas.

Every man should have people who can offer support in times of need. If you're the only one offering help in your circle of association, it's only a matter of time before you dry up. Having mentors who have accomplished the goals you have set out to achieve would help you achieve yours faster.

6. PRACTICE GRATITUDE

Gratitude is easy to ignore, especially when you're looking at big goals. Just as we discussed earlier, big goals take our eyes from small wins. It's easy to notice your shortcomings and miss recognizing your achievements along the way. This negativity can kill self-motivation. So remember to recognize the blessings in your life and the things you have accomplished so far.

Practice gratitude by taking note of what has happened that has worked and noticing positive changes no matter how small. Things might not be the way you want, but you're not where you used to be. I used to be terrible at savings, but now I have a clear savings system for my income. I used to be an easy quitter, but I've developed more grit.

A gratitude practice can help you feel proud of how far you've come while also teaching you the best ways to move forward. Cultivating the "attitude of gratitude" has proven benefits, too. These include inspiring self-motivation, opening the doors to new opportunities, and improving physical health (something you'll need to keep pushing ahead).

7. GET ENOUGH REST

If I stood on top of the Empire State Building and screamed this fact out, it still wouldn't be enough. Rest, rest, rest! To keep motivation strong, we must give ourselves time to pause and reset, especially during times of stress. Some people work themselves to exhaustion. Note exhaustion could be mental or physical. Physical exhaustion is easily noticeable, unlike mental exhaustion. At some point, you might feel like you can keep going, but never argue with your mind when it has had enough.

When I started running track in high school and college, I learned to eat before I felt hungry and drink before I felt thirsty. Taking care of yourself with breaks for relaxation will help sustain your motivation. And when you do hit a dip, rest helps you to be more resilient.

8. CELEBRATE ACHIEVEMENTS

Look back and use the perspective of miles completed as a means to give jet fuel into the tank for future moves. When hard work pays off, you absolutely deserve to celebrate and give yourself some credit. When you have a small win or reach a milestone on your journey, do whatever makes you feel like a superstar. That could mean taking time to yourself to walk on the beach, getting together with loved ones to celebrate, or treating yourself to a massage.

Remember, self-motivation is the art of pushing oneself to take initiative and action to pursue goals and complete tasks. By developing a general level of self-confidence in yourself, you will not only believe you can succeed, but you'll also recognize and enjoy the successes you've already had. That, in turn, will inspire you to build on those successes. The momentum created by self-confidence is hard to beat.

Having the self-motivation to set goals and work toward them takes a lot of hard work, and you deserve to reward yourself! Change doesn't happen overnight, but it's worth it! When you set out to achieve a big goal, expect to progress in small steps. When you feel a dip in self-motivation, remember all the concrete actions you can take to avoid crashing and giving up too soon. Turn to your friends, get guidance from wise people in your circle, practice self-care, and stay positive.

CHAPTER 8

EVOLVING IN MASCULINITY

PERSONAL GROWTH

Growth is a natural process of life. The existence of every living organism begins with conception then birth. Every man is born as a cute, cuddly baby, and with the passing of time and proper nurturing, he grows into full adulthood. Why are we on Earth if we don't grow? Growth is proof of life. I can't think of anything worse than a stagnant life without signs of growth and development.

Growth is first and foremost personal, and in the words of the famous author Leo Tolstoy, "Everyone thinks of changing the world but no one thinks of changing himself." If things must change in the environment around you, then it starts with you. Similar to everything in life, growth is a choice, you can choose to grow, and you can choose not to. But one thing you cannot choose are the consequences of your actions. If you are unwilling to grow, your results will lead to ruts and regrets.

Let me ask you a question real quick: What's positively different about who you are now and who you were, say, three weeks ago? If you had to think hard before coming up with a half-baked response, then probably nothing has changed about you. You're still courting your limitations and playing and embracing your fears. It's not enough to want to be a better man; you must do something about it. Successful and unsuccessful people don't differ much in terms of abilities. What sets them are apart are the desires they intentionally act upon.

FROM OCCASIONAL TO REGULAR

Once in a while, we stumble upon inspiration to do something differently and better. Then we enjoy brief stints of progress but lack the commitment to make it consistent. I'm not here to put you down or make you feel bad, but I want to encourage you. That model man you've always dreamed of becoming is attainable—that man who takes responsibility and overcomes setbacks and obstacles thrown in his path. Take a deep breath in and a deep breath out and say to yourself, "*I can do this.*" It's time for you to transcend from being an occasional learner to an intentional chaser of growth and progress. This is the path you've chosen today, and nothing will deter you.

THE SUCCESS TRAP

One of the greatest enemies of onward and continual success is the success of the past. Many times, we fall for the trap of reveling in past victories. We bask in the euphoria of past successes. I call this the **success trap!** You might be on the path of rebuilding your life and really not have much by way of achievements, or maybe you've had a few accomplishments. The point here is we must keep evolving in our masculinity by daring for more. The biggest room in the world is the room for improvement. The secret of longevity and relevance is to continually up your game.

PAST, PRESENT, AND FUTURE

Well there we have it. Now you know your past success can lull you into a state of mental inertia. You might get trapped in your comfort zone. Now we're moving on to the more common enemy of personal growth: past failures. Nothing stings more than reminiscing on the failures of the past. I've said the following words, "What were you thinking?" out loud when I've remembered some of the silly things I have done in the past. But we must learn to effectively manage the past and our present if we're going to have a bright future.

The past consists of previous events and happenings in your life, ones you could control and ones you could not control. Although they are in the past, these previous happenings can be so real and influential. It's important we learn how to handle our negative past so it doesn't hinder our chances of getting better. Here are some tips to effectively managing your past:

DON'T FEEL THREATENED BY FAILURE

The fiercest threat of failure is its effect on the mind. Ever heard of the term, "once a failure always a failure"? There's not a single shred of truth in this. Unfortunately, too many people tend to take this literally to the point where they start thinking they'll never succeed again. Such negative thoughts serve to do nothing but hold you back. This mind-set is so poisonous it leaves you crippled with fear of failure. Some people don't even bother trying because something keeps telling them they'll fail again. This mind-set will stand in the way of you reaching your full potential. If you're to move forward and lead a fulfilling life, you've got to overcome such stagnant thoughts and replace them with positive ones.

When we fail to accomplish our objectives, we increasingly become sensitive and uncomfortable, sometimes even over-whelmed with self-pity, disgrace, and outrage; this is how the average man responds to failure. Indeed, you could similarly say you feel hurt after a disappointment. Rather than being controlled by these feelings, use them for your potential benefit. Rather than feeling terrible and floundering in your pity party, let it drive you to work on a better future.

FOSTER HEALTHY HABITS TO STAY HEALTHY

In the event you haven't as of now started this practice: take strolls, work on breathing techniques, take a bath, and meet with loved ones—anything that keeps your mind clear and liberated from negative thoughts. Draw up a list of healthy habits and exercises you may like and put forth an attempt to rehearse them consistently. Who knows, one of these habits may even be the key to your prosperity!

In some cases, people take up using drugs or alcohol trying to numb the pain they feel. At last, they become junkies and alcoholics gradually, counting down to self-destruction. The euphoria of alcohol or substance abuse is only temporary, and the effects can cost you your life. Rather than going for a quick fix, develop and stick with healthy habits that will keep you healthy in the long run.

BE REASONABLY LIABLE FOR YOUR FAILURE

Imagining something somewhere is responsible for the way things turned out is counterproductive and an utter waste of time. In the same way, blaming everything on yourself will only leave you with feelings of anxiety and stress, which is pointless. Beating yourself up for past events will prevent you from learning from your errors. Try not to rationalize your disappointments. Put in effort to discover precisely why things went wrong, accept the role you had to play in it, and make corrections for the future.

STUDY YOURSELF

Many people feel disheartened after a failure while many others take failures as an opportunity to learn about and improve themselves. Where do you fit in? What mistakes have you made? In what areas are you lacking? By digging deep and learning about yourself, you're able to turn your failures into valuable life lessons and use the knowledge gained to achieve your goals.

KEEP LOOKING AHEAD

Don't get stuck focusing on the things that went wrong. Thinking about the same thing over and over again won't do you any good. While reflection on past failures is necessary, planning your next move and moving on is even more important.

TAKE INSPIRATION FROM FAILURES THAT LED TO SUCCESS

History is filled with stories of men and women who've all failed at some point in their lives but went on to become major successes in their respective areas. The one thing these people all had in common was they didn't let their failures stop them from experimenting and trying out new things. Learning about these people's past failures and how they overcame them can be a great source of inspiration for you to overcome your own shortcomings.

LEARN TO ACCEPT FAILURES

Fleeing from disappointments or attempting to stay away from them will do you no good. Go past your comfort zone and seek out new paths for yourself. Don't carry the thoughts of failure in your head but believe everything works for your good. As you push ahead every day in life, you will come to understand disappointment is just a normal part of life. The sooner you begin regarding failures as learning opportunities, the sooner you'll reach your maximum potential.

In case you're actually battling with disappointment and feel like nothing is happening for you, don't be hesitant to look for professional help. Regardless of how overpowered you may feel, always remember there are people out there devoted to help you to defeat failure and carry on with your personal business.

TAKING RESPONSIBILITY

Some college students once had the opportunity to question a successful and highly effective role model they loved. They said, "We find it hard to stay awake studying at night. And on some nights, we have to take NoDoz to stay awake. How do you manage such a busy schedule?" He smiled and said, "You take coffee to stay awake, I take responsibility!" A strong sense of responsibility for your life's outcome will help you make sacrifices.

Real men don't complain about their lives. They don't sulk when things go wrong. They keep pushing for something better. Evolving your masculinity means you have to gain mental, emotional, and financial independence. Mental independence is a state where you can think for yourself and make sound decisions. While growing up, we were subject to the decisions of our parents and guardians. Because we were still mentally underdeveloped, we had to trust their experience. But a time comes in every man's life when he has to decide what kind of man he wants to be and the kind of life he wants to live. It's up to you to build solid convictions. You must have a clear perspective on life and your definition of the relationships around you.

Next is emotional independence and maturity. Have you ever seen fully grown men with the emotional level of a teenager? There is a name for it I guess, a "man child." You must evolve your emotions. This doesn't mean you should shut down your feelings and become like a robot, but you must learn how to manage your emotions.

MANAGE YOUR EMOTIONS

Emotions are good, and they help us navigate through daily living, but if not properly managed, they will run us down. You need to get a hold of how you feel. Some people get deflated so easily anything can cause them to spiral into depression. Their self-motivation vanishes, and they find it hard to progress in life. Get a hold of your emotions!

Being emotionally stable also means you don't cry and bicker over every hurtful thing someone said to you. I saw a funny meme online that read, "If you don't want anyone to say anything negative to you, then go sell ice cream." In life, there will be people who may always speak ill of you; however, you must learn to deal with the situation. Whether you feel happy or sad, don't let it come in the way of your progress. Be in tune with your emotions but remember they are your emotions—yours to manage and control, not the other way around.

FINANCIAL RESPONSIBILITY

Finally, we come to financial independence. Money is an important tool in driving purpose. Money isn't everything, but it sure is something. Money in the right hands is a tool of great good, and in the wrong hands, a weapon of mass destruction. Every man ought to get to the point of financial independence. I'm not talking about having millions of dollars in your account or sipping expensive wine, but you must be able to pay your bills and afford yourself basic amenities like food, clothing, and shelter. If someone still pays your bills and gives you allowance, then you are not yet financially independent. The good news is anyone can make money in this time, whether he is a high school student, a school janitor, or the managing partner of a law firm. Anybody at all can make money. Gone are the days when you needed a diploma in finance and financing from a top business school in the state to be a big-time business guru.

According to a CNBC small business survey, less than half of people who make up the pool of business owners have a degree in business administration or marketing. They create the ideas and employ the first-class business degree holders to manage the resources. World-class author Robert Kiyosaki explains richness in his book that A students, more often than not, end up working for C students—an anomaly, right? It's an unpopular opinion that doesn't sit well with the old orthodox believer, but one that sadly is the truth (Kiyosaki, 2001).

Studying business management and having a job does not guarantee you a wealthy future; at most, you get a good retirement plan and a nice check for your service. The rules have changed. The world's richest today could be an IT analyst, a physicist, or a biochemist. How did they get there with little or no knowledge of how to handle their wealth? They employed the first-class business gurus. While they had time to pursue other interests, their money and their ideas kept making them more money. They pay you for your time and ideas in helping them grow their company while they search out other ways to build a better, bigger source of money channel. Like I said earlier, have a basic knowledge of whatever it is you intend to put your money into, and the rest can easily be sorted out.

A lot of people have businesses that have folded up even before they are launched because they place the insurmountable problem of creating capital before the main project itself. There are courses out there to learn how to earn from different streams of income: from real estate, to stocks, to cryptocurrency. If anybody can make money, how then does that happen? Why is the major part of the population not filled with wealthy millionaires? The answer can be found in the following:

- Knowledge (business mind-set)
- Passion
- Ideas
- Tenacity

Simple as they are, these are the ingredients to wealth creation. The only way to improve the quality of your life is to improve yourself.

Napoleon Hill was a self-help author of best-selling *Think and Grow Rich*. He said, "It's not what you are going to do, but it's what you are doing now that counts." Many unsuccessful people have what I call "someday sickness" because they could do some things to bring value to their lives right now but they put them off and say they'll do them someday. Their motto is "One of these days." But as the old English proverb says, "One of these days means none of these days." The best way to ensure success is to start growing today. No matter where you may be starting from, don't be discouraged; everyone who got where he is started where he was.

If you want to be a continual learner and keep growing throughout your life, you'll have to carve out the time to do it. You'll have to do what you can wherever you are. As Henry Ford said, "It's been my observation that most successful people get ahead during the time other people waste."

But growth is always worth the price you pay because the alternative is a limited lifetime of unfulfilled potential. Success takes effort, and you can't make the journey if you're sitting back waiting for life to come along and improve you. The future contains only what you put into it today. The seeds we sow in the present determines the harvest we will reap in the future. It's time to evolve into the best version of yourself.

CHAPTER 9

LEADERSHIP THROUGH SERVICE

There are thousands of books about leadership out there. I mean literally thousands of books providing great information on a panoramic view of leadership. Just a single Google search will reveal at least a half dozen titles about how to be a great leader: how to get people to listen to you, how to gain influence, and how to make a difference. You'll find titles about how to make your name known, build your company, or acquire positions of power.

Leadership isn't a new concept, and the world has for centuries raised great leaders who achieved remarkable feats and touched many lives. But when a man called Jesus came along, he decided to flip the narrative of leadership on its head. People didn't expect that at all. And it's not the kind of marketing strategy you'd find in a best-selling "how-to" leadership book today.

Jesus had a unique leadership philosophy, and it sure must have had heads spinning. This is what he said about leadership:

Jesus called them to Him and said, "You know how the kings of the nations show their power to the people. Important leaders use their power over the people. It must not be that way with you. But whoever wants to be great among you, let him care for you. Whoever wants to be first among you, let him be your servant. For the Son of Man came not to be cared for. He came to care for others. He came to give His life so that many could be bought by His blood and made free from the punishment of sin."

MATTHEW 20:25-28 (NLV)

This philosophy has been coined into a beautiful phrase: "servant leadership." The true goal of leadership is not grabbing power but service. Leadership isn't about making our names known. It's not self-seeking or self-preserving.

It's about service to God and humanity. We must serve people with love and respect. This is how a man should use his authority.

The concept of leadership is not limited to the traditional context of an organizational or social setting. Whether you're a CEO of an organization, the drum major of a high school marching band, a volunteer at church, or an older sibling everyone is leading someone. Knowingly or unknowingly, your actions have a great influence on someone. Someone is inspired by your life; someone is looking up to you for guidance and direction. I know this might be hard to believe, but it's true. Men all over the world can make a difference if we follow this truth. So how do you become a servant leader?

INTEGRITY

I put this first because it's the most important quality of a servant leader. The world is suffering so much from the misbehaviors of men who lack integrity. Countless relationships have been sunk for this reason: husbands cheating on their wives, fathers disappointing their children, or even employees not doing their best at work. Without integrity, we have nothing. It is the foundation on which all other leadership qualities are built. Proverbs 21:3 is a reminder Jesus calls us to walk in the ways of righteousness and justice; our actions should reflect our faith.

If we are true servant leaders, we can't cheat, lie, or manipulate our way to the top. We are called to do something much different and entirely countercultural—to be honest. It's sometimes difficult to stick to your morals when a lot of people are living life like they don't care. Without integrity, you'll be constantly adjusting to the standards of this world, injuring your conscience in the process.

The world tells us to do whatever it takes to achieve success and acclaim. Books tell us to dress and act a certain way to get noticed. Fairy tales tell us to just believe in ourselves. But without integrity, you can't effectively be a servant leader. What remains would be deception and manipulation.

Integrity is an intentional lifestyle, reflecting an overall track record of honesty and good character. We will stumble here and there, and we will fall short (because we're humans, after all). But true servant leaders can accept their shortcomings. There is a certain aura of reliability people of integrity carry. It's easier to trust someone true to his morals than a person who does whatever he wants without recourse to any moral standard. Another advantage is it helps you reach your fullest potentials because you are stable. You'll notice living by an integrity code will help you serve wholeheartedly. Your lifestyle will inspire people to want to do better. People become naturally drawn to you and you even become more confident.

Living life with integrity, especially in the face of challenges and temptations, is an incredible way to inspire and lead those who look up to us.

HUMILITY

So he got up from the table, took off his robe, wrapped a towel around his waist, and poured water into a basin. Then he began to wash the disciples' feet, drying them with the towel he had around him.

JOHN 13:4-5 NLT

One of the most difficult things to admit to ourselves and others is we don't know it all. It's common to see people try to always seem like they know it all. With the internet at the tip of our fingers, it can be tempting to swipe through a few pages in a search engine and convince ourselves we're an expert on a subject. It can be so easy to isolate ourselves in a bubble of self-knowledge and self-assurance, kicking out any and every opinion that doesn't align with what we want.

If we're not careful, we can become prideful. It's easy to become addicted to the power and authority attached to holding a leadership position. We meet and interact with different types of folks every day, at home, on the train, on a bus, or even at work, mask on or mask off in this post-COVID world. The best way to get the most out of a relationship is by simply being humble. I've met people desperately in need of help but their pride wouldn't let them ask.

Jesus, full of power and authority, was so humble as to bend down and wash the feet of his disciples; it takes so much confidence and contentment to have so much knowledge and power and yet be so humble.

A servant leader is someone who has built-in space to learn and grow from the experiences and opinions of others, so you're not just bossing people around.

In servant leadership, we have to be open to learn from and listen to those we lead because we know they have value and worth. The truth is they might actually have better ideas than we do or a perspective we don't. I have come to realize and accept my ideas are not the best and two heads are better than one.

Everyone has a story, a rich experience you could either ignore or learn from. But learning will be the better option of the two. When we listen to the stories of people, we begin to realize there are a lot of things we don't know. Being humble will expand your world's view. You'll begin to see its beauty and diversity, increasing your empathy and making you more approachable.

FLEXIBILITY

I know how to live on almost nothing or with everything. I have learned the secret of living in every situation, whether it is with a full stomach or empty, with plenty or little. For I can do everything through Christ, who gives me strength.

—PHILIPPIANS 4:1213 (NLT)

Servant leaders are very flexible people. They're willing to adapt to their situations and surroundings. Life is full of ups and downs. Things can change so quickly and leave you in a state of confusion. We must recognize life can throw us into unexpected situations or challenges. But instead of allowing those unexpected events to cause anger, confusion, or panic, servant leaders recognize they've been equipped to survive in every circumstance.

When you get used to a rigid way of doing things, it blinds you from seeing other possible solutions. Sometimes life sets obstacles on our path, but we must learn to maneuver around them. No problem is devoid of a solution; no case is too tough to crack. You must develop the willingness to practice being flexible, and positive changes will begin to take place.

It can be easy to get stuck in routines with one set way of doing things. But a servant leader's ability to recognize change for what it is—an opportunity for growth and faith—will help as they lead others well.

RESILIENCE

Tough times don't last, only tough people do. Resilience is the character and ability to stand your ground even in the face of troubles, offenses, and storms. If servant leadership were cheap and easy, everyone would be doing it. It is reserved for the big boys—those who have accepted a life of sacrifice. It takes a big heart to live, lead, and give sacrificially.

If you've ever trained for a race or played a sport, you know endurance doesn't just happen overnight. Initially, you have to trick your body into liking long distances! You run short distances first and build up to longer ones. You get blisters and you take water breaks, but eventually, you can run farther and longer. This works the same way in every aspect of life. No one all of a sudden becomes resolute and resilient. You must first practice it with the little things and move to larger things.

Resilient leaders can sustain their energy level under pressure to cope with disruptive changes and adapt. They bounce back from setbacks. They also overcome major difficulties without engaging in dysfunctional behavior such as **people-pleasing, constantly feeling guilty, having poor communication skills, and feeling empty and isolated**. Resilience is a crucial characteristic of high-performing leaders. Leaders must cultivate it in themselves to advance and thrive. They also carry the responsibility of helping protect the energy of the people in their teams. Leadership is sustainable only if individuals and teams are able to consistently recover high energy levels.

Nelson Mandela is a great example of resilience. He was sent to prison as a young freedom fighter who believed in taking up means of resistance when the justice system failed. Twenty-seven years later, he came out advocating peace and reconciliation. During his long confinement, Mandela mastered the art of self-leadership. He took great inspiration in the poem "Invictus" written by William Ernest Henley, which ends with the verses "I am the master of my fate / I am the captain of my soul."

Life will always have challenges: fights we cannot win, mountains we just can't climb, and dark valleys with no visible way out. Resilience in the Christian life can only happen when we look to Jesus.

During life's challenges, God's constant presence is our source of comfort. Our higher power doesn't always fix our circumstances, and sometimes the solution isn't on our timetable, but God will always help us get through it with love, strength, patience, and more.

Servant leaders recognize struggles are real and life is difficult, but God is in control. Resilience isn't an absence of fear, challenges, or momentary failures. Resilience is the ability to bounce back, to push through, and to press on based on the truth God has enabled us to persevere because divine energy is our ultimate source of strength.

STEWARDSHIP

As each has received a gift, use it to serve one another, as good stewards of God's varied grace.

—1 PETER 4:10 (ESV)

People's minds tend to go straight to money when they think of stewardship, but it goes beyond managing money. One of Merriam-Webster's definitions of the word is "the careful and responsible management of something entrusted to one's care." The first thing we should note is everything you have was given to you. This helps you avoid being proud and cocky.

We've been gifted with unique abilities and gifts. Could you imagine what life would be like if everyone thought, looked, and acted the same? Life would be so dull! What will make life even more pleasant is when we use these gifts to bless others. This is the definition of true leadership.

Unfortunately, this concept seems so hard to grasp these days. Most men assume controlling roles in the lives of the people they lead. They may say, "I pay the bills around here, so you better do whatever I say." In the same way, some bosses believe paying their employees a good wage gives them the ability to mistreat them.

To get the best from people, you must engage them openly and lovingly. People tend to know when a person is genuinely interested in their growth and development.

So while being good stewards of our finances is definitely something, we should also learn to steward other things of value, such as our purpose, talents, friendships, and relationship with our higher power.

A servant leader sees people as valuable to God and stewards their time and talents well. This kind of leader calls out what is good and true about the people they lead, giving them instruction and encouragement in how to serve God well. A servant leader uses their time for God's glory, not their own.

Lead by example. A good leader wouldn't ask you to do something they would be unwilling to do themselves. When this kind of person interacts with you, you'll know it. You'll leave interactions feeling like you are valued and your talents are being leveraged for a greater cause. That's an example worth following!

EMPATHY

Be happy with those who are happy, and weep with those who weep.

—ROMANS 12:15 (NLT)

Empathy is the ability to emotionally understand what other people feel, see things from their point of view, and imagine yourself in their place. Essentially, it is putting yourself in someone else's position and feeling what they must be feeling. When you see another person suffering, you might be able to instantly envision yourself in the other person's place and feel sympathy for what they are going through.

While people in general can show empathy, getting into someone else's head can be a bit more difficult. The ability to feel empathy allows people to "walk a mile in another's shoes," so to speak. It plunges you into the emotions others are feeling.

Many people may not comprehend seeing someone in pain and responding with indifference or even outright hostility. But the fact some people do respond in such a way clearly demonstrates empathy is not an ability everyone has.

How many times have you had a friend or family member sit with you when you were hurting? Have you ever received an encouraging note from someone when you needed it most?

Think about what it meant for you to have a person truly empathize with you during your struggles.

Empathy is a key aspect of leadership. It's easy to get hyper-focused on the tasks and work we do. Work is important, and accomplishing goals is too! But if we're not careful, we can begin to see people as problems to be solved instead of human beings to be loved.

Some signs that show you tend to be an empathetic person:

- You are good at really listening to what others have to say.
- People often tell you about their problems.
- You often think about how other people feel.
- You are good at picking up on how other people are feeling.
- Other people come to you for advice.

- You often feel overwhelmed by tragic events.
- You are good at telling when people aren't being honest.
- You try to help others who are suffering.
- You sometimes feel drained or overwhelmed in social situations.
- You care deeply about other people.
- You find it difficult to set boundaries in your relationships with other people.

Empathy allows people to build deep connections with others. By understanding what people are thinking and feeling, people can respond appropriately in social situations. Research has shown having social connections is important for both physical and psychological well-being.

Empathizing with others helps you learn to regulate your own emotions. Emotional regulation is important in that it allows you to manage what you are feeling, even in times of great stress, without becoming overwhelmed.

Empathy promotes servant leadership. Not only are you more able to direct people but you also feel empathy for them.

Not everyone experiences empathy in every situation. Some people may be more naturally empathetic in general, but people also tend to feel more empathetic toward some people and less so toward others.

Some of the different factors that play a role in this tendency include:

- How people perceive the other person

- What people attribute the other individual's behaviors to
- What people blame for the other person's predicament
- Past experiences and expectations

A servant leader can see people through the eyes of Jesus. That's the kind of leader that others follow!

When we're able to take time out of our day to empathize with those around us and put ourselves in their shoes, we become more like Jesus. Whenever Jesus encountered someone who was hurting or in need of encouragement, he looked at them and had compassion for them. Then he acted.

Leadership might seem intimidating. A lot of responsibility goes into it. But servant leadership also brings the potential to witness to others and demonstrate Jesus in ways other positions wouldn't have fully allowed. Focusing on the ideas mentioned in this chapter, such as **integrity, humility, flexibility, resilience, stewardship, and empathy,** allows you to build trust with those around you, and ultimately the people around you are inspired by your actions. Take some time today to think about the people in your life God is calling you to lead. And when it's time to make decisions within that role, ask yourself a famous question: "What would Jesus do?"

CONCLUSION

——

WHAT IS THE TAKEAWAY?

The journey of life is full of twists and turns. Sometimes life slams us down so hard it's a tough call getting back up. But all this contention takes place in the mind. Mental health is a serious thing, and it's important as men, we practice self-care. Self-care is not selfishness; in fact, it shows we love people. If you get swallowed up by disorders and mental illness, you won't be of much help to the ones you love and the world at large. This is such an important practice. The same way we take baths and groom our bodies, we also can groom our minds.

There are no limitations to how far we can go. We can build solid relationships with our family, friends, and business partners. Money is not the greatest resource a man can have, people are. It takes wisdom to cultivate and maintain solid and healthy relationships—relationships where we partner with each other for growth and development. We must have people who we can be ourselves with and people who urge us to be better.

If we ask ourselves the right questions, we'll have a better insight into the happenings in our lives. It also helps us heal and move forward, even as we find purpose. A man is said to have not lived until the day he discovers his purpose. Just like pirates hunt for treasure, we must diligently seek out our purpose. Knowing your purpose gives life a fresh sense of meaning and direction. Making decisions becomes easier because you can put it through the purpose test. Every day when you wake, practice self-motivation and don't wait for anyone to give you a pep talk. Learn to push yourself even when you don't feel like it, and learn to rest and refresh your energies.

We have discussed tips to build solid relationships and mental wholeness and deal with trauma. Throughout the book, healing through self-examination can lead to finding your purpose and motivation. Ultimately, I want to help you grow as a person who is an emotionally strong, effective communicator who values your mental health and wellness. The advice given throughout the book shows all of us have the ability to grow at our own pace. We want to grow to support not only ourselves but our loved ones around us.

It was Henry Ford who said, "If you say you can you're right, if you say you can't, you're also right." The ball is in your court; you can take a shot at your goals or sit idle doing nothing. But our idle days are long gone. Having read this book, I leave you with a passionate heart ready to take over your world. Take a leap of faith and grow.

ACKNOWLEDGMENTS

Thank you.

I want to start by saying thank you to those of you who read this. Your eyes passing over these words means the world and more to me.

Most of all, I want to thank God for grace and mercy—the source of strength on my journey.

My family has also seen my evolution. I love you all, and thank you for being the support system within the support system. My parents Michael Sr and Esther, my sibling Stephen. My uncles, aunts, cousins, and extended family. To Janna. Thanks for being my cool ex-wife. To Lailah and Charles, or should I say my motivation and inspiration to be a good dad? I love y'all.

My oldest friends Shawn, Sherwin, Sheldon Thwaites, Chris and TnT Steelpan family, Mike George and Caiso Steelband, Rick, Toussaint, Derek, I C Gray aka Dan Appleget, Ron Blocker, Jason, Kenny A, Dan, Stephen, Padmore, Dr. Jack, Mike Bobo, Dr. Gadson, William, Daria, Kristi, Brady, Craig, Andre, Coach Chris, Coach Roger, Coach Pam, Tim,

Shannon and save the day Ray, George, Thomas, Sonya, Jason & Tamika, Orin. To the Brothers of Alpha Phi Alpha, incorporated, Mighty Mu Rho chapter, Full Speed Athletic track family. Towson University & Howard University, respectively. To my mentors Bro Erik King, Bro Jean, Bro Willie, Elder Otis, Elder Thomas, James Livingston, Dr Buckingham, Bro Charles Motte, Dr. White-Hood, Principal Clowers, distinguished Toastmasters LaMonica and Beverly. Thanks for sharing your wisdom with me, the best is yet to come. Thank you all so much, your love and support mean the world.

To Adrienne, your energy is amazing, I'm grateful God guided our paths to align; you inspire me.

To Bashae, Niketa, and Monroe, it's a pleasure working with Hearts in Mind counseling.

I'm a proud Eagle Scout representing troop 1656. We were Black Excellence in the Boy Scouts led by Bruce Beuzard, Mr. Vines, Mr. Mateen, Mr. Epperson, and Ms. Brasfield. Thank you for teaching us to always give 110 percent, to my Wild at Heart and Prayer line Bros. I appreciate you a lot.

Mike Max, Kenny O, Noel we are "Alliance of Destiny" Thank you for being their during my most challenging moments, keeping it real with me at all times. Love y'all Bros.

To Professor Koester: thank you for encouraging me. Your dedication to helping students become writers is a divine gift.

To Coach Desmond Dunham: Congrats on your book "Running Against the Odds" and thank you for telling me about the Book Creator Institute. We beat the odds and became published authors. Thanks for all you do for the youth.

To NDP staff, especially Whitney, Chuck, and Venus: thank you for making this book a reality and working with me.

To Mario Armstrong and the Never Settle family, we are entrepreneurs from all walks of life let's keep chasing our dreams. To Phil Lampron, the Softball Hall of Fame and renowned photographer. To Thomas Pollard, Tony Jackson, and Cliff Exil thanks for the encouragement over the years. I appreciate you guys more than you know.

To past professors, teachers, mentors, and coaches who always encouraged me: thank you for seeing what you did in me. It still means the world today.

To all of those who contributed to my IndieGoGo Campaign and those whose words of encouragement from start to finish I consider priceless. A heartwarming thank you for being early supporters of Tribe of Men, the book.

APPENDIX

INTRODUCTION

"Infographic for Men's Mental Health." Mental Health America. Accessed January 13, 2021.

MEN NEED SELF-CARE TOO

Bruce, Debra. "Exercise and Depression." WebMD. February 2020. https://www.webmd.com/depression/guide/exercise-depression

Bryne, Rhonda. *The Secret*. New York: Atria books, 2006.

MENTAL WHOLENESS

Anthenelli, Robert and Lindsey Grandison. "Effects of Stress on Alcohol Consumption," Alcohol Res. 34, no. 4 (2012): 381–382. https://www.ncbi.nlm.nih.gov/pmc/articles/PMC3860387/#!po=85.0000.

Bryne, Rhonda. *The Secret*. New York: Atria books, 2006.

Soul Salt. "Conversational Intelligence®: A Path to Effective Leadership." Accessed September 25, 2021. https://soulsalt.com/conversational-intelligence/.

DEALING WITH TRAUMA

Kessler, Ronald C. et al. "Trauma and PTSD in the WHO World Mental Health Surveys." *European Journal of Psychotraumatology* 8, sup5 1353383. October 27, 2017, doi:10.1080/20008198.2017.1353383.

Lifelenscounseling. "Chronic Trauma." https://lifelenscounseling.com/chronic-trauma/.

Leonard, Jayne and Timothy Legg (eds). "What to Know About Alexithymia." MedicalNewsToday. Accessed September 25, 2021.

National Center for PTSD, "Anger and Trauma." https://www.ptsd.va.gov/understand/related/anger.

US Center for Substance Abuse Treatment. "Understanding The Causes Of Trauma." Trauma-informed Care in Behavioral Health Services. (United States: Rockville(MD), 2014) TIP series, No.57.

FINDING PURPOSE

Gordan, Mara. "What's Your Purpose? Finding A Sense of Meaning in Life Is Linked To Health." NPR. May 25, 2019. https://www.npr.org/sections/health-shots/2019/05/25/726695968/

whats-your-purpose-finding-a-sense-of-meaning-in-life-is-linked-to-health.

Warren, Rick. *Purpose Driven Life: What on Earth Am I Here For?* Grand Rapids: Zondervan, 2002.

THE ART OF SELF-MOTIVATION

Boyatzis, Richard. Harvard Business Review, HBR Idea cast, Episode 699: What Great Coaching Looks Like, September 2019. https://hbr.org/podcast/2019/09/what-great-coaching-looks-like

Deci, Edward. *Intrinsic Motivation.* New York: Plenum Press, 1975.

Duckworth, Angela. *Grit: The Power of Passion and Perseverance.* New York: Scribner Publishers, 2016.

Glaser, Judith. *Conversational Intelligence: How Great Leaders Build Trust and Get Results.* London: Routledge, 2016.

Goldman, Daniel, J. Davidson et al. *Emotional Self Awareness: A Primer,* (Florence, MA: More Than Sound LLC, 2017)

Nagoski, Emily and Amelia Nagoski. *Burnout: The Secret to Unlocking the Stress Cycle.* New York: Random House Publishing Group.

Soul Sault. "How to Believe in Yourself (in 5 simple steps)." Accessed September 25, 2021, https://soulsault.com/how-to-believe-in-yourself/.

Stajkovic, A.D. and F. Luthans. "Self Efficacy and Work Related Performance: A Meta-analysis." *Psychological Bulletin* 124 (1998): 240–261.

Wang, Q., Timberlake, M. A., Prall, K., and Dwivedi, Y. "The recent progress in animal models of depression." *Progress in Neuro-Psychopharmacology & Biological Psychiatry* 77 (2017): 99–109. https://doi.org/10.1016/j.pnpbp.2017.04.008

EVOLVING IN MASCULINITY

Juang, Mike. "A Secret Many Small-Business Owners Share with Mark Zuckerberg." CNBC. July 19, 2017. https://www.cnbc.com/2017/07/19/survey-shows-majority-of-business-owners-lack-college-degree.html.

Kiyosaki, Robert and Sharon Letcher. *Rich Kid, Smart Kid: Giving Your Child A Financial Headstart.* Plata Publishing, 2001.

LEADERSHIP THROUGH SERVICE

Shipp, Lydian. "The Most Common Dysfunctional Family Characteristics, How To Spot Them, And What Can Be Done." Regain. April 21, 2021. https://www.regain.us/advice/family/the-most-common-dysfunctional-family-characteristics-how-to-spot-them-and-what-can-be-done/.

Made in the USA
Middletown, DE
19 March 2023

27110041R00070